To
Cathy and Greg Caswell

CONTENTS

LIST OF TOPICS & ILLUSTRATIONS

Text: One page of text is devoted to each of the following topics. *Illustrations are listed in italics.*

PREFACE

An Illustrated Review of Anatomy and Physiology is a series of ten books written to help students effectively review the structure and function of the human body. Each book in the series is devoted to a different body system.

My objective in writing these books is to make very complex subjects accessible and unthreatening by presenting material in manageable size bits (one topic per page) with clear, simple illustrations to assist the many students who are primarily visual learners. Designed to supplement established texts, they may be used as a student aid to jog the memory, to quickly recall the essentials of each major topic, and to practice naming structures in preparation for exams.

INNOVATIVE FEATURES OF THE BOOK

(1) Each major topic is confined to one page of text.

A unique feature of this book is that each topic is confined to one page and the material is presented in outline form with the key terms in boldface or italic typeface. This makes it easy to scan quickly the major points of any given topic. The student can easily get an overview of the topic and then zero in on a particular point that needs clarification.

(2) Each page of text has an illustration on the facing page.

Because each page of text has its illustration on the facing page, there is no need to flip through the book looking for the illustration that is referred to in the text ("see Figure X on page xx"). The purpose of the illustration is to clarify a central idea discussed in the text. The images are simple and clear, the lines are bold, and the labels are in a large type. Each illustration deals with a well-defined concept, allowing for a more focused study.

PHYSIOLOGY TOPICS (1 text page : 1 illustration)
Each main topic in physiology is limited to one page of text with one supporting illustration on the facing page.

Anatomy Topics (1 text page : several illustrations)
For complex anatomical structures a good illustration is more valuable than words. So, for topics dealing with anatomy, there are often several illustrations for one text topic.

(3) Unlabeled illustrations have been included.

In Part II, all illustrations have been repeated without their labels. This allows a student to test his or her visual knowledge of the basic concepts.

(4) A Pronunciation Guide has been included.

Phonetic spellings of unfamiliar terms are listed in a separate section, unlike other textbooks where they are usually found in the glossary or spread throughout the text. The student may use this guide for pronunciation drill or as a quick review of basic vocabulary.

(5) A glossary has been included.

Most textbooks have glossaries that include terms for all of the systems of the body. It is convenient to have all of the key terms for one system in a single glossary.

ACKNOWLEDGMENTS

I would like to thank the reviewers of the manuscript for this book who carefully critiqued the text and illustrations for their effectiveness: William Kleinelp, Middlesex County College; and Robert Smith, University of Missouri, St. Louis, and St. Louis Community College, Forest Park. Their help and advice are greatly appreciated. Kay Petronio is to be commended for her handsome cover design and Bob Cooper has my gratitude for keeping the production moving smoothly. Finally, I am greatly indebted to my editor Bonnie Roesch for her willingness to try a new idea, and for her support throughout this project. I invite students and instructors to send any comments and suggestions for enhancements or changes to this book to me, in care of HarperCollins, so that future editions can continue to meet your needs.

Glenn Bastian

An Illustrated Review of the CARDIOVASCULAR SYSTEM

1 The Heart

1

HEART / Overview of the Cardiovascular System

HISTORICAL BACKGROUND

William Harvey (one-way blood flow)

In 1628 William Harvey, an English physician, demonstrated that blood flows in one direction through blood vessels, and thus discovered that blood circulates (the *circulatory* system). Prior to this time it was believed that blood flowed out of the heart and back into the heart by way of the same vessels, like the tide's ebb and flow. The evidence for this assumption was based on anatomical dissection. It was clear to anatomists that the large vessels attached to the heart branched into smaller and smaller vessels and finally ended in the organs. But since microscopes had not yet been invented, it was not possible to see the small microscopic vessels that connected the large branches, forming loops or circuits.

Marcello Malpighi (capillaries)

It was not until late in the 17th century that Marcello Malpighi, an Italian physiologist, observed capillaries through his microscope, and thus discovered the anatomical link between arteries (the vessels carrying blood away from the heart) and veins (the vessels carrying blood toward the heart). Malpighi's discovery supported by direct observation what Harvey had concluded by deductive reasoning.

CIRCULATORY ROUTES

Blood vessels are organized into parallel routes that carry blood throughout the body. There are two basic routes : the pulmonary circulation and the systemic circulation.

Pulmonary Circulation (the right heart)

The right heart (right ventricle) pumps blood to the lungs, where oxygen is absorbed and carbon dioxide is released. From the lungs the freshly oxygenated blood is carried to the left atrium. This short loop is called the pulmonary circulation.

Systemic Circulation (the left heart)

The left heart (left ventricle) pumps oxygenated blood to all the tissues of the body. Oxygen and nutrients are released from the blood to nourish the cells; carbon dioxide and metabolic wastes are collected and carried to the lungs and kidneys where they are excreted.

DISTRIBUTION OF BLOOD

Within the systemic circulation there are minor circuits arranged in parallel that carry blood to each organ of the body. Arteries carry blood away from the heart to organs; veins carry blood back to the heart from the organs. Most of the blood pumped by the left heart goes to one of six major organs : brain, heart, kidneys, skeletal muscle, gastrointestinal (GI) tract, and skin.

Under normal circumstances (at rest) each ventricle of the heart pumps about 5 liters of blood per minute; this is known as the cardiac output. In the systemic sytem, the blood is distributed between the major organs : 3/4 liter to the brain, 1/4 liter to the heart muscle, 1 1/2 liters to the gastrointestinal (GI) tract, 1 liter to the kidneys, 1 liter to the skeletal muscles, and 1/2 liter to the skin. After a meal a greater proportion of the blood goes to the GI tract; during physical exercise a greater proportion of the blood goes to the skeletal muscles. The amount of blood to the brain is constant at all times.

(For simplicity, the illustration on the facing page omits the circuit to the heart.)

CARDIOVASCULAR SYSTEM OVERVIEW
Pulmonary Circulation : gray shading
Systemic Circulation : white

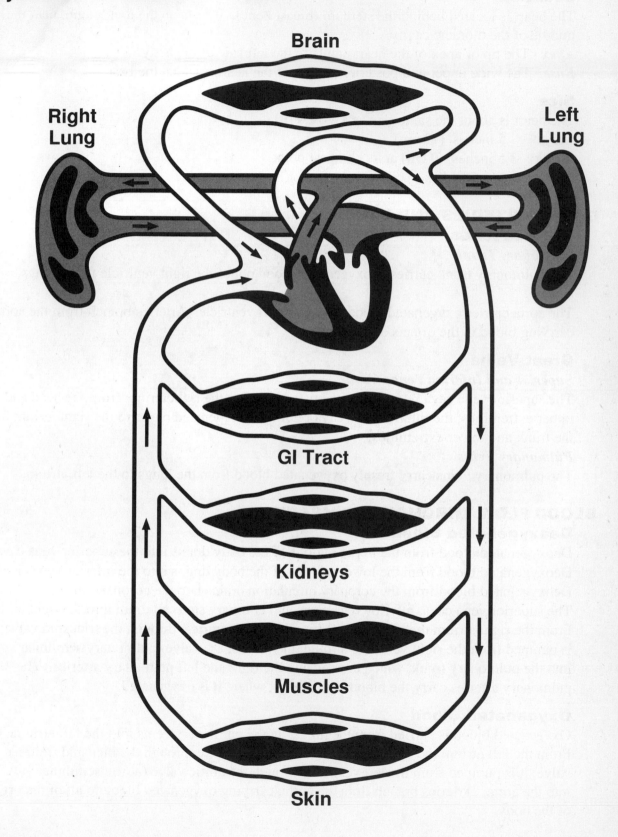

Brain

Right Lung

Left Lung

GI Tract

Kidneys

Muscles

Skin

HEART / Superficial Anatomy

LOCATION AND SIZE
Location
The heart is located behind the sternum (breast bone). It rests on the diaphragm, near the middle of the thoracic cavity.

Apex The tip or apex of the heart points to the left side of the body.

Base The wide upper and posterior margin of the heart is called the base.

Size
The heart is about the same size as a closed fist.

Length : 5 inches (12 cm).

Width : 3.5 inches (9 cm) at its broadest point.

Thickness : 2.5 inches (6 cm).

GREAT ARTERIES AND VEINS
Great Arteries
Pulmonary Trunk

The pulmonary trunk carries deoxygenated blood out of the right ventricle to the lungs.

Aorta

The aorta carries oxygenated blood out of the left ventricle. Arteries branch from the aorta, carrying blood to the organs of the body.

Great Veins
Superior and Inferior Venae Cavae

The superior vena cava returns deoxygenated blood to the right atrium from the head and upper extremities; the inferior vena cava returns deoxygenated blood to the right atrium from the trunk and lower extremities.

Pulmonary Veins

The pulmonary veins carry freshly oxygenated blood from the lungs to the left atrium.

BLOOD FLOW THROUGH THE HEART
Deoxygenated Blood
Deoxygenated blood from the upper regions of the body drains into the superior vena cava. Deoxygenated blood from the lower regions of the body drains into the inferior vena cava. Deoxygenated blood from the coronary circulation drains into the coronary sinus.

The superior vena cava, inferior vena cava, and coronary sinus all drain into the right atrium. From the right atrium the blood passes into the right ventricle through the tricuspid valve; it is pumped from the right ventricle through the pulmonary valve (pulmonary semilunar valve) into the pulmonary trunk, which divides into the right and left pulmonary arteries. The pulmonary arteries carry the blood to the lungs, where it is oxygenated.

Oxygenated Blood
Oxygenated blood is carried from the lungs via the pulmonary veins into the left atrium. From the left atrium the blood passes into the left ventricle through the bicuspid (mitral) valve; it is pumped from the left ventricle through the aortic valve (aortic semilunar valve) into the aorta. Arteries branch from the aorta, carrying oxygenated blood to all of the organs of the body.

HEART ANATOMY
Superficial Anterior View

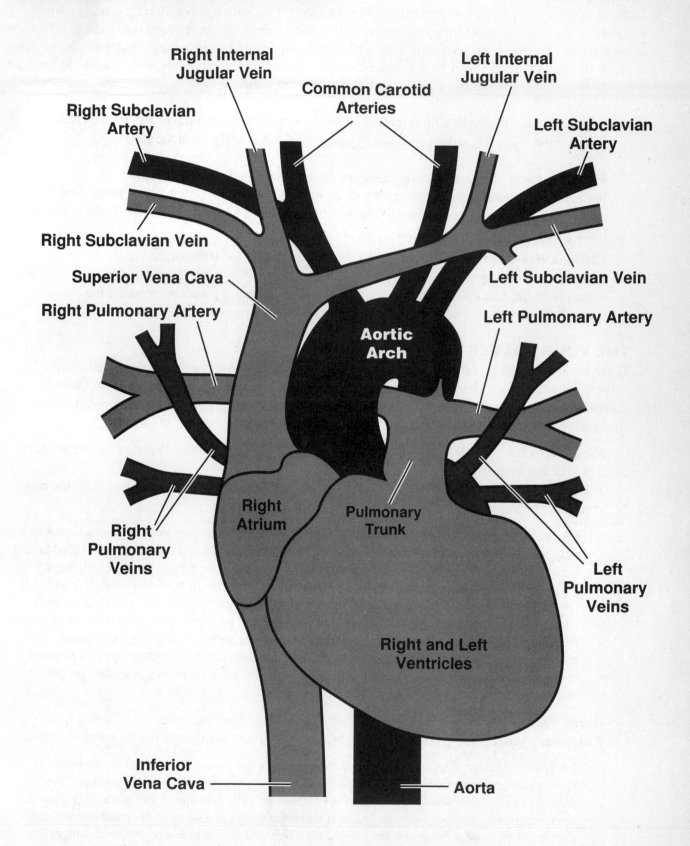

Right Internal
Jugular Vein

Common Carotid
Arteries

Left Internal
Jugular Vein

Right Subclavian
Artery

Left Subclavian
Artery

Right Subclavian Vein

Left Subclavian Vein

Superior Vena Cava

Left Pulmonary Artery

Right Pulmonary Artery

Aortic
Arch

Right
Pulmonary
Veins

Right
Atrium

Pulmonary
Trunk

Left
Pulmonary
Veins

Right and Left
Ventricles

Inferior
Vena Cava

Aorta

HEART / Chambers and Valves

THE FOUR CHAMBERS

There are four separate spaces or chambers in the heart. Two atria receive blood returning to the heart via the veins; two ventricles act as muscular pumps, which squeeze blood out of the heart into the arteries. The ventricles have thick muscular walls capable of creating the pressure needed to push blood through the blood vessels; the muscular walls of the atria are relatively thin, since little force is required to squeeze blood from an atrium into its adjacent ventricle.

Right Atrium   The right atrium receives deoxygenated blood from the organs of the body.
Left Atrium   The left atrium receives oxygenated blood directly from the lungs.

Right Ventricle   The right ventricle pumps deoxygenated blood to the lungs.
It generates a maximum pressure at rest of 25 mm Hg (mercury). The highly elastic tissues of the lungs offer little resistance to blood flow and the distance the blood must travel is short, so the force generated is relatively small.

Left Ventricle   The left ventricle pumps oxygenated blood to all the organs of the body.
It generates a maximum pressure at rest of about 120 mm Hg. It has a muscular wall thicker and more powerful than the right ventricle, since it requires greater pressure to propel the blood through the extensive system of tubes that carries blood throughout the body.

THE FOUR VALVES

There are four one-way valves in the heart. The atrioventricular valves (bicuspid and tricuspid valves) connect atria with their adjacent ventricles; the semilunar valves (pulmonary and aortic valves) connect ventricles with their great arteries. All valves open and close in response to pressure changes on either side.

Bicuspid Valve (Left AV Valve or Mitral Valve)   The bicuspid valve separates the left atrium from the left ventricle. It is composed of two flaps of tissue.
Tricuspid Valve (Right AV Valve)   The tricuspid valve separates the right atrium from the right ventricle. It is composed of three flaps of tissue.

Chordae Tendineae   The AV valves must be very flexible since they must be pushed open by a very small force—the pressure gradient between the atrial blood and the ventricular blood is less than 1 mm Hg. At the same time, they must be very strong to withstand the relatively high pressures of the blood that push against them during contraction of the ventricles. If it were not for the tendons (called chordae tendineae) attaching these valves to the inner walls of the ventricles, they would evert (turn inside out), and there would be a reflux of blood back into the atria.
Papillary Muscles   Papillary muscles located on the inner surface of the ventricles regulate the tension in the chordae tendineae. When the ventricles contract, the papillary muscles contract also; this tightens the chordae tendineae and prevents the valve cusps from everting (turning inside out) into the atria.

Aortic Valve   The aortic valve separates the left ventricle from the aorta.
Pulmonary Valve   The pulmonary valve separates the right ventricle from the pulmonary trunk.

Backflow of Blood   The valves between the ventricles and great arteries prevent the backflow of blood into the ventricles. After blood is ejected from the heart, the ventricles relax and the pressures in the ventricular spaces drop very suddenly. The pressure in the aorta and pulmonary artery drop also, but more slowly. Almost immediately the pressures in the great arteries exceed the pressures in their corresponding ventricles. This shift in the pressure gradient changes the direction of blood flow. It flows back toward the heart, but is blocked by the one-way valves.

HEART ANATOMY
Chambers and Valves

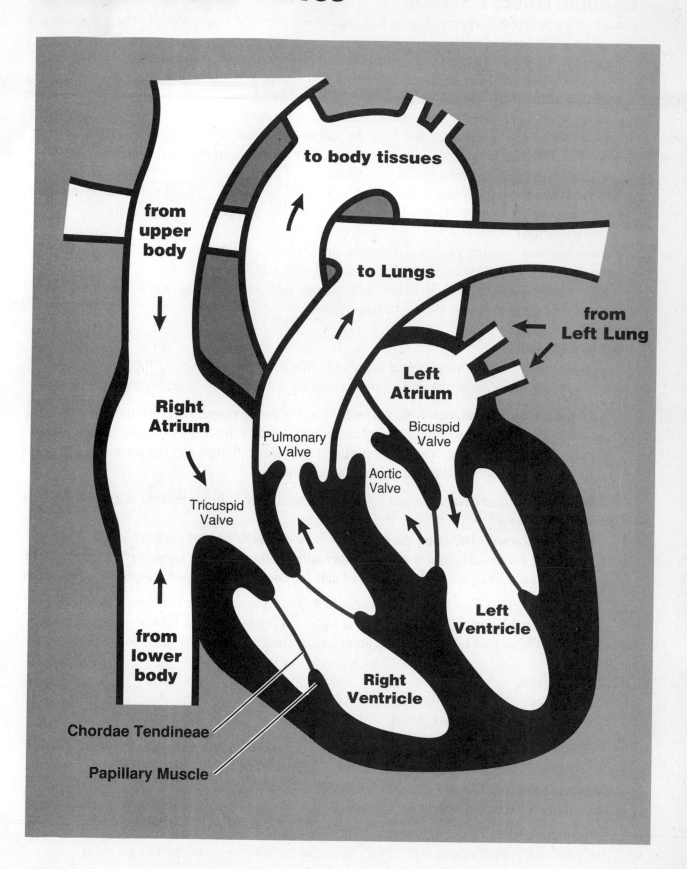

to body tissues

from upper body

to Lungs

from Left Lung

Right Atrium

Left Atrium

Pulmonary Valve

Bicuspid Valve

Aortic Valve

Tricuspid Valve

Left Ventricle

from lower body

Right Ventricle

Chordae Tendineae

Papillary Muscle

HEART / Tissues

CARDIAC MUSCLE TISSUE

Cardiac muscle tissue consists of branched, cylindrical, striated fibers (cells), which contain one or two centrally located nuclei.

Branched Fibers   The branching structure allows the cardiac muscle fibers to form networks. When one fiber is electrically excited, the impulse (action potential) is quickly transmitted to the neighboring fibers that make up the network. Thus, an impulse spreads in all directions as it moves throughout cardiac muscle tissue.

Intercalated Discs   Intercalated discs are unique to cardiac muscle; they are irregular transverse thickenings of plasma membrane (sarcolemma) between attached heart muscle cells. They contain desmosomes and gap junctions.

Desmosomes   Desmosomes act as reinforcing spot welds; their function is to hold adjacent cells together.   They are located on the lateral borders of adjacent muscle cells.

Gap Junctions   Gap junctions are small channels filled with cytoplasm; their function is to allow impulses (action potentials) to pass quickly between neighboring cells. They are located on the terminal borders of adjacent muscle cells.

Filaments   In cardiac muscle fibers the filaments (actin and myosin) are not packaged in myofibrils (as they are in skeletal muscle fibers).

PERICARDIUM

The pericardium is the double-layered membrane that surrounds the heart. It is formed by the invagination (pushing in) of the pericardial sac during the 4th week of embryonic development.

Fibrous Pericardium (outer layer)   The fibrous pericardium is a tough membrane composed of heavy fibrous connective tissue that protects the heart from overdistension during vigorous exercise. The lower portion rests on the diaphragm; the upper portion fuses with the great vessels entering and leaving the heart.

Serous Pericardium (inner layer)   This relatively delicate portion of the pericardium consists of a double layer.

Parietal Layer   The outer parietal layer is fused to the fibrous pericardium.

Visceral Layer   The inner visceral layer adheres tightly to the muscle of the heart. It is considered to be part of the heart wall and for this reason it is also called the *epicardium*.

Pericardial Cavity   The pericardial cavity is a small space between the parietal and visceral layers of the serous pericardium. It contains a thin film of serous fluid that holds the two layers together and reduces friction caused by heart movements.

HEART WALL

Three layers form the wall of the heart : the epicardium (external layer), myocardium (middle layer), and endocardium (inner layer).

Epicardium   The epicardium (or visceral layer of the serous pericardium) is the thin, transparent membrane surrounding the heart. It is attached to the myocardium.

Myocardium   The myocardium is the thick portion of the heart wall, consisting of myofibers (cardiac muscle cells).

Endocardium   The endocardium is the inner lining of the heart. It consists of endothelial cells and is continuous with the lining of the great vessels attached to the heart.

TISSUES

Cardiac Muscle

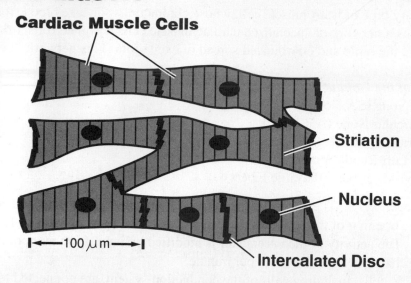

Cardiac Muscle Cells

Striation

Nucleus

|← 100 μm →|

Intercalated Disc

Pericardium and Heart Wall

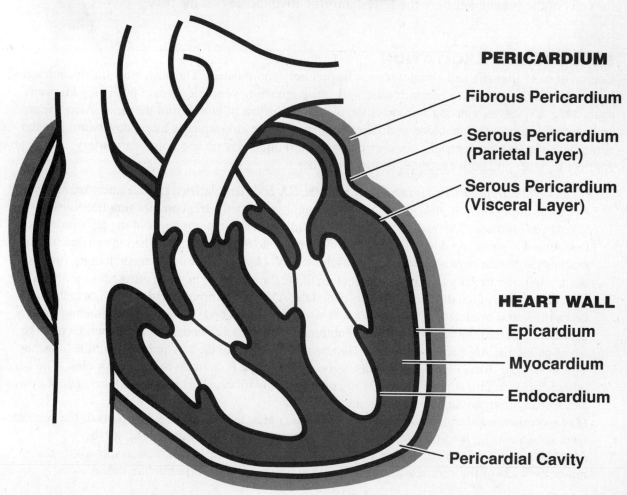

PERICARDIUM

Fibrous Pericardium

Serous Pericardium
(Parietal Layer)

Serous Pericardium
(Visceral Layer)

HEART WALL

Epicardium

Myocardium

Endocardium

Pericardial Cavity

HEART / Conduction System

STRUCTURES

Besides the ordinary type of heart muscle cell, whose contractions squeeze blood from the chambers of the heart, there is a network of specialized cardiac muscle cells designed for starting each heart contraction and for the rapid and coordinated spread of excitation. This network of cells is called the conduction system.

Components of the Conduction System
(1) Sinoatrial Node (SA Node or Pacemaker)
(2) Atrioventricular Node (AV Node)
(3) Atrioventricular Bundle (AV Bundle or Bundle of His)
(4) Right and Left Bundle Branches
(5) Conduction Myofibers (Purkinje Fibers)

SA Node (Pacemaker)   The cells of the pacemaker (a small mass of cells embedded in the right atrial wall near the opening of the superior vena cava) depolarize spontaneously at a rate of 100 times per minute. The activity of the pacemaker is modified by input from autonomic nerves, so at rest the rate of discharge is about 75 times per minute.

All heart muscle cells, including cells of the conduction system, are connected to each other by cytoplasmic strands called *gap junctions*. These gap junctions make it easy for electrical impulses to spread between adjacent cells. So, immediately after a heart cell depolarizes, the cells around it depolarize. In this manner a wave of excitation and contraction spreads over the entire heart. Since the cells of the pacemaker have the fastest intrinsic rhythm, they set the pace.

SEQUENCE OF EXCITATION

Contractions of the atria and ventricles must be precisely coordinated. The atria must finish contracting before the ventricles start to contract; otherwise, the contracting ventricles would push blood upward against the AV valves, causing them to close, blocking the flow of blood from the atria. Also, the atria and ventricles must squeeze blood in different directions—the atria squeeze blood downward into the ventricles, whereas the ventricles squeeze blood upward into the aorta and pulmonary artery. (Both atria contract together and both ventricles contract together.)

(1) SA Node Depolarizes   Immediately after the SA node depolarizes, special fibers rapidly carry electrical impulses from the right to the left atrium, so that both atria contract simultaneously.
(2) Atria Contract   The wave of excitation spreads from the upper regions of the atria downward; thus, blood is squeezed down through the AV valves into the ventricles. When the electrical impulse reaches the border between atria and ventricles it is blocked by a band of nonconducting fibrous tissue. In order to get past this nonconducting tissue the electrical impulse must pass through a specialized area of small-diameter fibers called the AV node (atrioventricular node), which slows down the speed of electrical transmission. This delay (0.1 second) gives the atria time to finish contracting before the ventricles begin to contract. The AV node connects with a bundle of large fibers called the AV bundle (bundle of His), which divides into the left and right bundle branches. This system of fibers carries the impulse very rapidly to the bottom tip of both ventricles. The bundle branches divide into smaller fibers called conduction myofibers (Purkinje fibers) that radiate upward and spread throughout the ventricular muscle.
(3) Lower Ventricular Muscle Contracts   The heart muscle cells in the lower parts of the ventricles contract, squeezing the blood upwards, pushing open the pulmonary and aortic valves.
(4) Middle and Upper Ventricular Muscle Contracts   The wave of contraction spreads up the muscular walls of the ventricles, squeezing blood into the aorta and pulmonary artery.

CONDUCTION SYSTEM

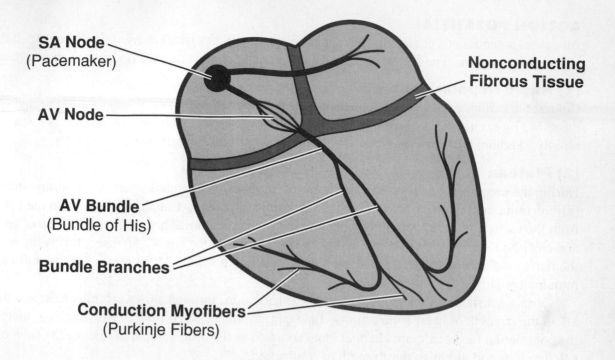

SA Node
(Pacemaker)

Nonconducting
Fibrous Tissue

AV Node

AV Bundle
(Bundle of His)

Bundle Branches

Conduction Myofibers
(Purkinje Fibers)

Sequence of Excitation
Regions of excitation in black

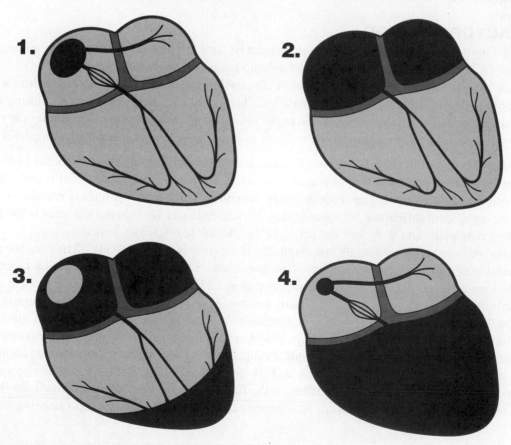

1.

2.

3.

4.

HEART / Cardiac Muscle Contraction

ACTION POTENTIAL
An action potential is a change in the membrane potential (electrical charge) of a muscle cell that triggers contraction. The action potentials of contractile cardiac muscle fibers have three phases.

(1) Rapid Depolarization   *Voltage-gated fast Na⁺ channels open.*
Contractile cardiac muscle fibers have a resting potential of -90 mV. When they are brought to threshold by excitation in neighboring fibers, voltage-gated fast sodium (Na^+) channels open very rapidly. Sodium ions rush into the cells, producing a rapid depolarization.

(2) Plateau   *Voltage-gated slow Ca²⁺ channels open.*
During the second phase, voltage-gated slow calcium (Ca^{2+}) channels open in the plasma membrane (sarcolemma) and the membrane of the sarcoplasmic reticulum. Calcium diffuses into the cytosol from the extracellular fluid and from the sarcoplasmic reticulum. The combined buildup of sodium and calcium ions in the cytosol maintains the depolarization for about 250 msec; this is the reason for the horizontal section (plateau) on the graph of an action potential. In contrast, skeletal muscle fibers remain depolarized for only 1 msec.

Certain substances alter the movement of calcium ions through slow Ca^{2+} channels, and thus affect the strength of heart contractions. Epinephrine enhances the flow of calcium ions, increasing the contraction force; calcium channel blockers, such as the drug verapamil, reduce the flow of calcium ions and diminish the strength of contraction.

(3) Repolarization   *Voltage-gated K⁺ channels open.*
During repolarization, potassium (K^+) channels open and potassium ions diffuse out of the cell into the extrcellular fluid. At the same time, the Na^+ and Ca^{2+} channels are closing. The resting membrane potential of -90 mV is restored, and the muscle fiber relaxes.

REFRACTORY PERIOD
The refractory period of cardiac muscle is significant because it prevents the heart from seizing up. If the heart were to seize up, like a clenched fist, it could no longer pump the blood.

Refractory means unresponsive or stubborn. In physiology it refers to the period of time when a muscle or nerve cell is unresponsive to stimulation. There are two refractory periods : during the *absolute* refractory period a cell will not respond regardless of how strong the stimulus; during the *relative* refractory period a cell will respond if the stimulus is suprathreshold (stronger than a threshold stimulus).

Cardiac Muscle vs. Skeletal Muscle   The absolute refractory period for muscle cells lasts approximately as long as the muscle action potential. As soon as the muscle action potential is completed, a suprathreshold stimulus can trigger another action potential, which causes a muscle response (contraction). One significant difference between cardiac muscle cells and skeletal muscle cells is the length of their action potentials, and therefore the length of their absolute refractory periods.

Cardiac muscle action potentials last about 250 milliseconds (0.25 second). The time for contraction and relaxation of cardiac muscle is about 300 milliseconds. So the cardiac muscle action potential is almost as long as its period of contraction and relaxation. This means that the cardiac muscle cell cannot start to contract a second time until it has nearly completed its relaxation period. This is extremely important, because it is during the period of ventricular relaxation that the heart fills with blood; if it doesn't have time to properly fill, it will have less blood to pump, decreasing the cardiac output.

Skeletal muscle action potentials last only 1 millisecond. The time for relaxation and contraction of a skeletal muscle cell is about 150 milliseconds. This means that a skeletal muscle cell can be stimulated to contract again before it has had time to relax. If the frequency of stimuli is great enough the skeletal muscle cell will go into a state of sustained contraction (tetanus), as when a weight is being held.

ACTION POTENTIALS
Cardiac Muscle Compared to Skeletal Muscle

Cardiac Muscle

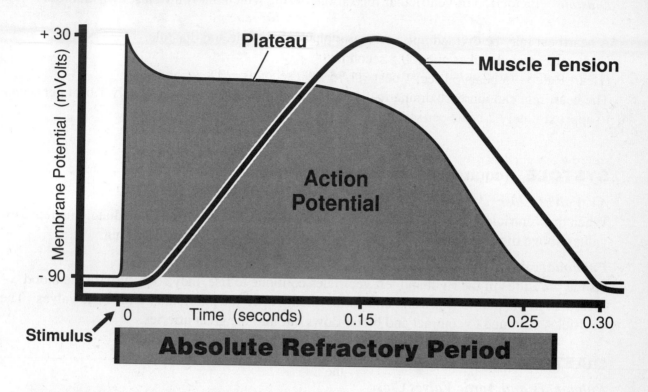

Plateau

Muscle Tension

Action Potential

Membrane Potential (mVolts)

+30

-90

Stimulus

0   Time (seconds)   0.15   0.25   0.30

Absolute Refractory Period

Skeletal Muscle

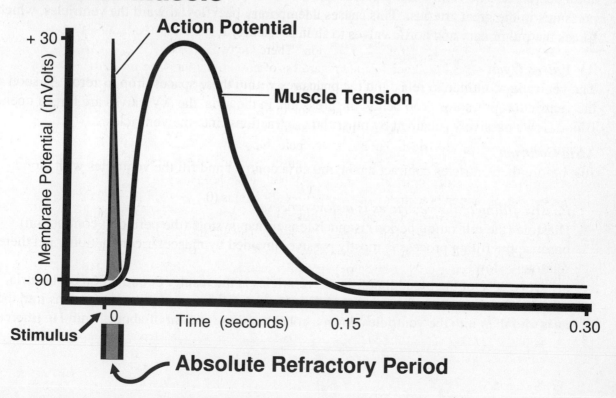

Action Potential

Muscle Tension

Membrane Potential (mVolts)

+30

-90

Stimulus

0   Time (seconds)   0.15   0.30

Absolute Refractory Period

13

HEART / Cardiac Cycle : Systole and Diastole

Cardiac Cycle : all of the events associated with one heartbeat.
Systole : the period of ventricular contraction and blood ejection.
Diastole : the period of ventricular relaxation, during which the ventricles fill with blood.

A heartbeat may be divided into two major phases : systole and diastole.
Each cardiac cycle takes about 0.8 second.
(Heart Rate = 75 beats/60 sec; 1 beat = 1/75 x 60 seconds = 0.8 second.)
The heart rate can increase dramatically during exercise—from approximately 1 beat per second to approximately 2 beats per second.

SYSTOLE   (contraction) 0.3 second

AV Valves Close
When the ventricles contract, the blood pressures inside the ventricles immediately increase to values above the pressures in the atria. Consequently, the AV valves snap shut.

Pulmonary and Aortic Valves Open
As the pressures in the right and left ventricles continue to rise, they soon surpass the blood pressures in the pulmonary trunk and aorta, forcing open the pulmonary and aortic valves. The ventricles continue to contract and blood flows out into the great arteries.

DIASTOLE   (relaxation) 0.5 second

Pulmonary and Aortic Valves Close
As the ventricles relax, the pressures in the ventricular spaces and in the pulmonary trunk and aorta decrease. The ventricular pressures drop more rapidly and soon they are less than the pressures in the great arteries. This causes a temporary backflow toward the ventricles, which forces the pulmonary and aortic valves to shut.

AV Valves Open
The ventricles continue to relax and the pressures within these spaces drop to zero. As soon as the ventricular pressures drop below the pressures in the atria, the AV valves are forced open. Blood flows passively (unaided by muscular contractions) into the ventricles.

Atria Contract
Just before the ventricles contract again, the atria contract and fill the ventricles with blood.

> *Passive filling of the ventricles is a slow process.*
> Diastole (the relaxation period) is much longer than systole (the period of contraction), because the filling process is mostly passive (unaided by muscular contraction), and therefore relatively slow.
>
> Only 20% of the blood that fills the ventricles is the result of contraction of the atria. The other 80% flows passively and slowly from the venae cavae and pulmonary veins into the atria and then into the ventricles down a concentration gradient of about 1 mm Hg (mercury).

SYSTOLE AND DIASTOLE

Ventricles contract.
Blood is ejected into the great arteries.

Systole

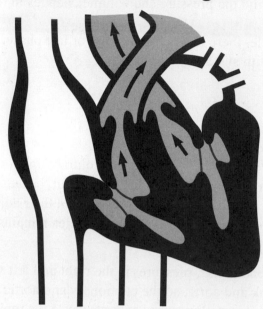

Ventricles relax.
Blood flows into the ventricles from the atria.

Diastole

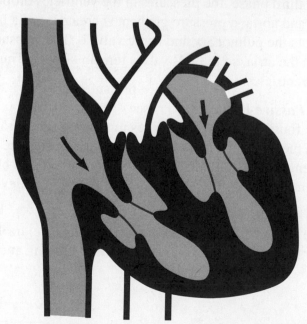

HEART / Cardiac Cycle : The Five Phases

A heartbeat may be divided into two phases, systole and diastole, but the complexity of a heartbeat can be understood more precisely by subdividing systole into two phases and diastole into three phases. The resulting five phases of the cardiac cycle are based on the opening and closing of the heart valves and the pressure and volume changes in the ventricles, atria, aorta, and pulmonary trunk.

Since it is a cycle, there is no absolute first or last phase. The illustration on the facing page arbitrarily begins with systole.

SYSTOLE

Phase 1 : Isovolumetric Contraction
During the first phase, the ventricles are contracting, but there is no blood flow out of the heart. The pulmonary and aortic valves are shut, because the pressures in the pulmonary trunk and aorta are greater than the pressures in their adjoining ventricles. Isovolumetric means that the volume of blood in the ventricles remains constant.

Phase 2 : Ejection
During the second phase, pressures in the right and left ventricles surpass the pressures in the pulmonary trunk and aorta, so the pulmonary and aortic valves are forced open. Blood is ejected from the heart. Pressure gradients cause the movement of blood that pushes open the pulmonary and aortic valves.

DIASTOLE

Phase 3 : Isovolumetric Relaxation
During the third phase, the pressures in the ventricles drop below the pressures in the pulmonary trunk and aorta; a pressure gradient is created, and a brief backflow of blood in the great arteries shuts the pulmonary and aortic valves. The pressure in the ventricles remains higher than that in the atria, so the AV valves remain closed. Thus, there is no blood flow into or out of the ventricles.

Phase 4 : Passive Filling
During the fourth phase, the pressures in the ventricles drop to zero, making them slightly lower than the pressures in their adjoining atria, which are about 1 mm Hg. The small pressure gradient is enough to push open the AV valves, and blood flows slowly from the atria into the ventricles. 80% of the ventricular filling is achieved by this passive flow of blood.

Phase 5 : Atrial Contraction
During the fifth phase, the atria contract, forcing an extra 10 ml of blood into each ventricle. This occurs just before the ventricles contract, starting another cardiac cycle.

CARDIAC CYCLE : The Five Phases

1 Isovolumetric Contraction

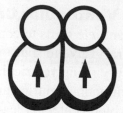

2 Ejection

Systole

3 Isovolumetric Relaxation

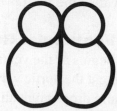

4 Passive Filling

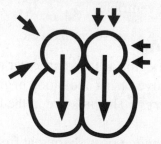

Diastole

5 Atrial Contraction

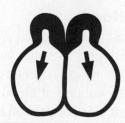

HEART / Cardiac Cycle : Pressure and Volume Changes (in the Left Ventricle)

Phase 1 : Isovolumetric Ventricular Contraction

AV Valve Shuts   Just after the ventricle starts to contract, the increased blood pressure in the ventricle forces the bicuspid (mitral) valve to shut.

Ventricular Pressure   The steeply rising ventricular pressure curve reflects the increasing muscle tension created by the contracting ventricular muscles.

Blood Volume (no change)   No blood enters or leaves the ventricles during the first phase, since both valves—the bicuspid valve and the aortic valve—remain closed.

Phase 2 : Ejection

Aortic Valve Opens   At the start of the second phase, the ventricular pressure curve intersects with the aortic pressure curve, and the aortic valve opens, allowing blood to flow from the left ventricle into the aorta.

Ventricular and Aortic Pressure   The ventricular and aortic pressures are the same throughout the second phase.

Blood Volume   The blood volume of the left ventricle drops sharply from 130 ml to about 60 ml as blood is ejected. The volume of blood left in a ventricle following its systole is called the *end–systolic volume (ESV)*, which is equal to 60 ml in this case. The amount of blood ejected from a ventricle during systole is called the *stroke volume (SV)*, which in this case is 70 ml.

Phase 3 : Isovolumetric Ventricular Relaxation

Aortic Valve Closes   This phase begins as the ventricular pressure curve intersects with the aortic pressure curve. At this moment the aortic valve snaps shut.

Aortic Pressure   The aortic pressure drops gradually, as pressure is dissipated in the system.

Ventricular Pressure   The ventricular pressure drops sharply as the ventricle relaxes.

Blood Volume   Since the aortic and bicuspid valves are both closed, there is no movement of blood into or out of the the left ventricle.

Phase 4 : Passive Filling

AV Valve Opens   This phase begins as the ventricular pressure curve intersects with the atrial pressure curve; the bicuspid valve opens and blood begins to flow into the ventricle.

Atrial and Ventricular Pressures   The pressure in the left atrium is slightly greater than that in the left ventricle.

Blood Volume   The volume change rises sharply at first and then levels off as the pressure gradient decreases.

Phase 5 : Atrial Contraction

This phase begins as the atrium contracts, squeezing an additional 10 ml of blood into the left ventricle. Both the atrial and ventricular pressure curves rise slightly at this time, as additional blood is forced into the left ventricle by atrial contraction.

End-diastolic Volume (EDV)   The volume of blood remaining in a ventricle at the end of its relaxation phase (just before ventricular contraction begins) is called the end-diastolic volume. At rest, it is about 130 ml.

CARDIAC CYCLE
Pressure and Volume Changes

Pressure Changes in the Left Ventricle

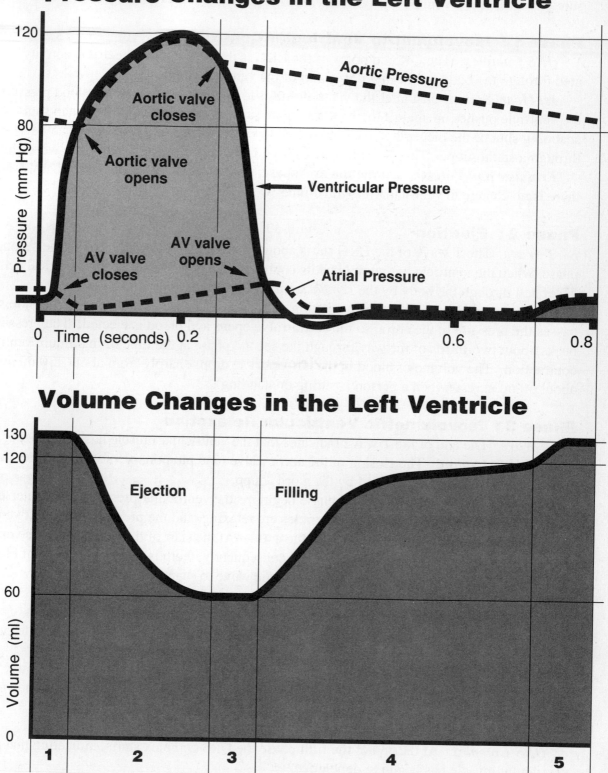

Aortic valve closes

Aortic Pressure

Aortic valve opens

Ventricular Pressure

AV valve closes

AV valve opens

Atrial Pressure

Pressure (mm Hg)

120

80

0   Time (seconds)   0.2   0.6   0.8

Volume Changes in the Left Ventricle

Ejection

Filling

Volume (ml)

130
120

60

0

1   2   3   4   5

HEART / Cardiac Cycle : Summary

The graph on the facing page illustrates the events that occur in the left ventricle during two cardiac cycles. It shows the relationship between electrical activity (EKG), heart sounds, pressure changes, blood volume changes, and the five phases of the cardiac cycle.

Phase 1 : Isovolumetric Ventricular Contraction

QRS Complex The QRS complex of the EKG is the result of the electrical activity generated through the body by the *depolarization* of the ventricular muscle.

1st Heart Sound Just after the ventricle starts to contract, the increased blood pressure in the ventricle pushes up against the bicuspid valve (mitral valve), causing it to snap shut. The snapping shut of the bicuspid valve (and tricuspid valve) causes vibrations that can be heard through a stethoscope. This is the first heart sound, and it is characterized by the word "lubb."

Pressure and Volume During the first phase, the ventricular pressure rises sharply, but there is no change in ventricular blood volume.

Phase 2 : Ejection

T Wave The T wave of the EKG starts about two-thirds of the way through the second phase, when the ventricle has completed its contraction; it is the result of the electrical activity generated through the body by the *repolarization* of the ventricular muscle cells.

Pressure and Volume At the beginning of the second phase the ventricular pressure surpasses the pressure in the aorta, so the aortic valve opens and blood is ejected. The pressure peaks about two-thirds of the way through the second phase at the time of maximum ventricular contraction. The volume of blood in the left ventricle drops sharply from about 130 ml down to about 60 ml at rest (when a person is sitting or standing).

Phase 3 : Isovolumetric Ventricular Relaxation

T Wave The end of the T wave indicates that the ventricular muscle has repolarized.

2nd Heart Sound The closing of the aortic valve (and pulmonary valve) generates the second heart sound, characterized by the word "dupp."

Pressure and Volume The third phase begins as the ventricular pressure curve intersects with the aortic pressure curve. The ventricles are relaxing, and the pressure in the left ventricle drops more suddenly than the pressure in the aorta. At the start of the third phase the ventricular pressure drops below the aortic pressure; consequently, there is a brief backflow of blood in the aorta toward the heart, which forces the aortic valve to snap shut.

Phase 4 : Passive Filling

P Wave The P wave of the EKG is the result of the electrical activity generated through the body by the depolarization of the atrial cells. This occurs just before the atria contract.

Pressure and Volume This is the longest phase. About 60 ml of blood flows slowly and passively (no musclular contraction) from the pulmonary veins into the left atrium and ventricle.

Phase 5 : Atrial Contraction

QRS Complex At the end of the fifth phase the QRS complex starts, indicating that the ventricular muscle has begun to depolarize.

Pressure and Volume Atrial contraction forces about 10 ml of additional blood into the left ventricle.

CARDIAC CYCLE : Summary

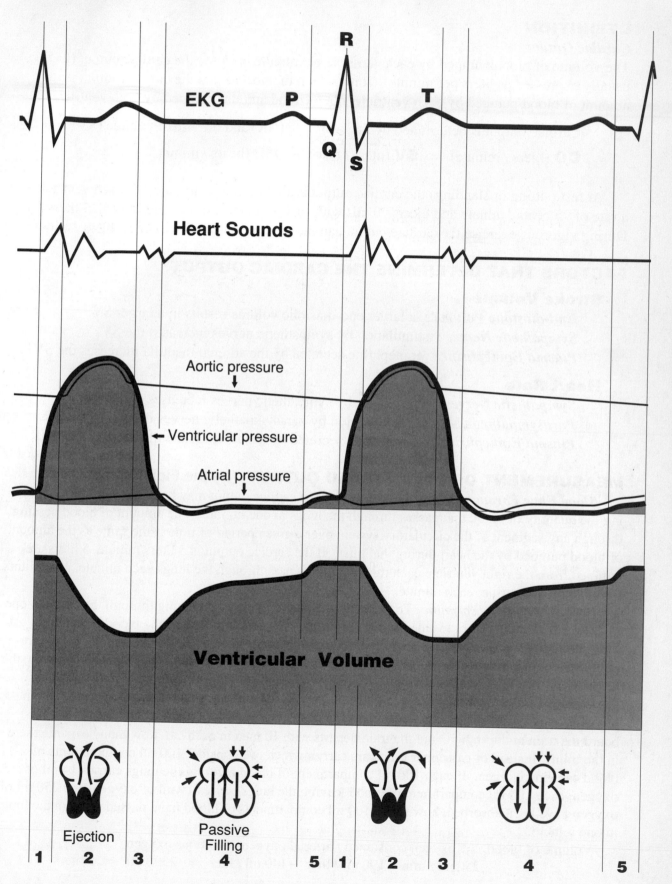

EKG

P

R

Q

S

T

Heart Sounds

Aortic pressure

← Ventricular pressure

Atrial pressure

Ventricular Volume

Ejection

Passive Filling

1 2 3 4 5 1 2 3 4 5

HEART / Cardiac Output : Overview

DEFINITION

Cardiac Output

The volume of blood pumped by each ventricle per minute is called the cardiac output (CO), usually expressed as liters per minute. (It must be remembered that the cardiac output is the amount of blood pumped by <u>each</u> ventricle, not the total amount pumped by both ventricles.)

Cardiac output is determined by the heart rate (HR) and the stroke volume (SV) :

CO (liters / minute) **= SV** (liters / beat) **X HR** (beats / minute)

At rest (sitting or standing) the cardiac output is about 5 liters / minute. If each ventricle has a rate of 75 beats / minute and ejects 70 mL with each beat, the cardiac output is 5.25 liters / min. During vigorous exercise the cardiac output can increase 6 or 7-fold to 30 or 35 liters / minute.

FACTORS THAT DETERMINE THE CARDIAC OUTPUT

Stroke Volume

End-diastolic Volume : a larger end-diastolic volume results in a larger SV.
Sympathetic Nerves : stimulation by sympathetic nerves increases the SV.
Plasma Epinephrine : epinephrine secreted by the adrenal medulla increases the SV.

Heart Rate

Sympathetic Nerves : stimulation by sympathetic nerves increases the HR.
Parasympathetic Nerves : stimulation by parasympathetic nerves decreases the HR.
Plasma Epinephrine : epinephrine secreted by the adrenal medulla increases the HR.

MEASUREMENT OF THE CARDIAC OUTPUT (by the Fick Method)

Blood Flow Through the Lungs (ml/min) The cardiac output may be determined by calculating the quantity of blood that passes through the lungs in one minute. The amount of blood passing through any segment of the circulatory system over a given period of time is the same as the amount of blood pumped by the heart during that time. If the cardiac output is 5 liters/minute, 5 liters are pumped from the right ventricle each minute, 5 liters pass through the lungs each minute, and 5 liters return to the left atrium each minute.

Rate of Oxygen Absorption To calculate the quantity of blood passing through the lungs in one minute, it is first necessary to calculate the amount of oxygen absorbed by the blood per minute. At rest 250 ml of oxygen are absorbed by the blood per minute. By comparing the oxygen concentration of the blood *entering* the lungs with the oxygen concentration of the blood *leaving* the lungs, the volume of blood passing through the lungs can be determined.

Passenger Train Analogy The passenger train analogy is sometimes used to make this math problem easier to visualize. If a passenger train enters a station with 5 men in each car, 100 men board the train at the station, and the train departs with 10 men in each car, how many cars are there in the train? Instead of passenger train cars carrying men, we consider 100 ml compartments of blood carrying oxygen. If each 100 ml compartment of blood entering the lungs carries 14 ml of oxygen, each 100 ml compartment of blood leaving the lungs carries 19 ml of oxygen, and 250 ml of oxygen have been absorbed, how many 100 ml compartments of blood have passed through the lungs in one minute?

Volume of blood = oxygen consumed / arterial oxygen − venous oxygen
250 ml / min ÷ 190 ml / liter − 140 ml / liter = 250 / 50 = 5 liters

CARDIAC OUTPUT
Factors That <u>Increase</u> the Cardiac Output

↑ Cardiac Output = ↑ Stroke Volume X ↑ Heart Rate

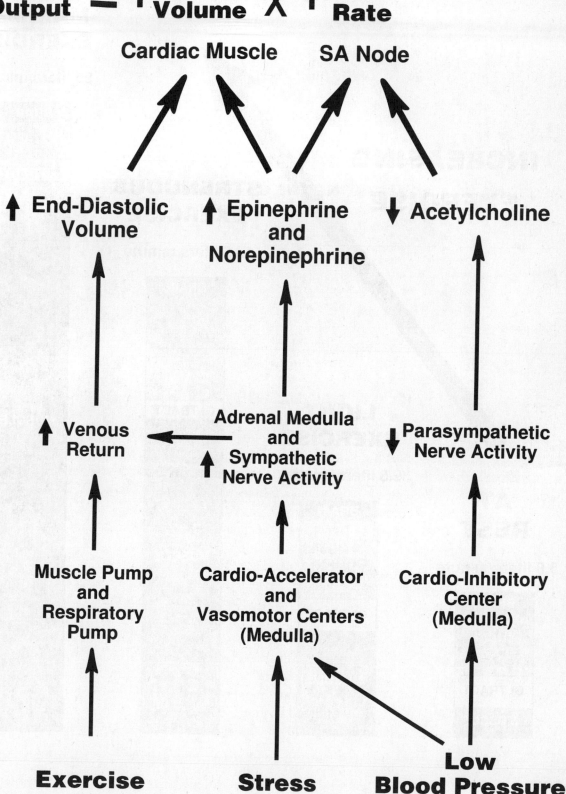

Cardiac Muscle   SA Node

↑ End-Diastolic Volume   ↑ Epinephrine and Norepinephrine   ↓ Acetylcholine

↑ Venous Return   Adrenal Medulla and ↑ Sympathetic Nerve Activity   ↓ Parasympathetic Nerve Activity

Muscle Pump and Respiratory Pump   Cardio-Accelerator and Vasomotor Centers (Medulla)   Cardio-Inhibitory Center (Medulla)

Exercise   Stress   Low Blood Pressure

CARDIAC OUTPUT
Effect of Exercise on CO and Blood Distribution

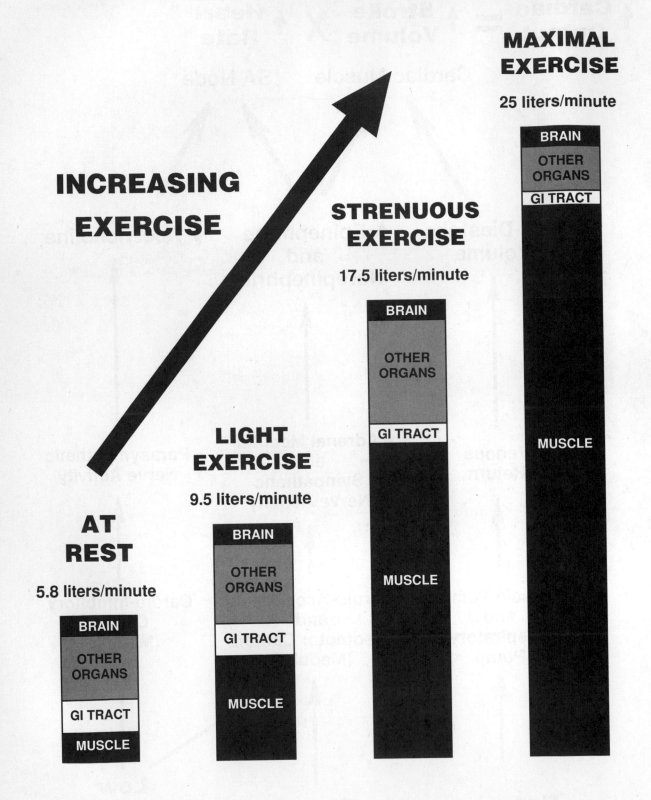

INCREASING EXERCISE

MAXIMAL EXERCISE

25 liters/minute

- BRAIN
- OTHER ORGANS
- GI TRACT
- MUSCLE

STRENUOUS EXERCISE

17.5 liters/minute

- BRAIN
- OTHER ORGANS
- GI TRACT
- MUSCLE

LIGHT EXERCISE

9.5 liters/minute

- BRAIN
- OTHER ORGANS
- GI TRACT
- MUSCLE

AT REST

5.8 liters/minute

- BRAIN
- OTHER ORGANS
- GI TRACT
- MUSCLE

CARDIAC OUTPUT
Measured by the Fick Method

The Passenger Train Analogy

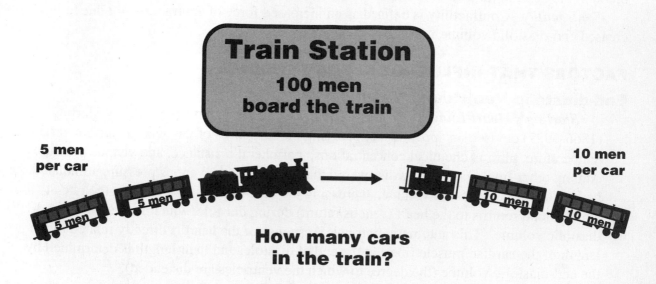

Train Station

100 men
board the train

5 men
per car

5 men

5 men

10 men
per car

10 men

10 men

How many cars
in the train?

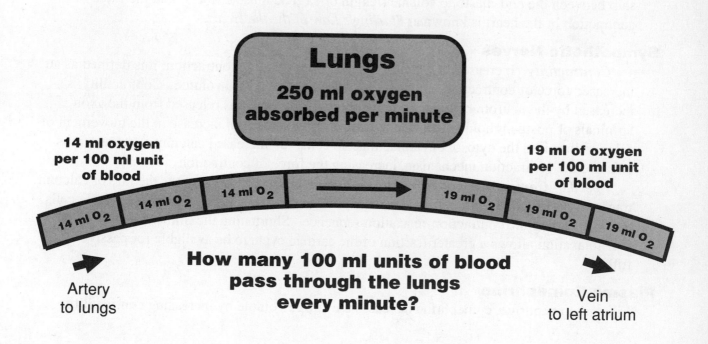

Lungs

250 ml oxygen
absorbed per minute

14 ml oxygen
per 100 ml unit
of blood

14 ml O₂   14 ml O₂   14 ml O₂

19 ml of oxygen
per 100 ml unit
of blood

19 ml O₂   19 ml O₂   19 ml O₂

Artery
to lungs

How many 100 ml units of blood
pass through the lungs
every minute?

Vein
to left atrium

HEART / Cardiac Output : Stroke Volume

DEFINITIONS

Stroke Volume   The stroke volume is the volume of blood ejected by a ventricle during a single contraction. The stroke volume at rest is about 70 ml.

End-diastolic Volume   At rest, each ventricle contains about 130 ml of blood when filled. This is the amount of blood in the ventricle just before ejection. Because this is the amount of blood in the heart at the end of the diastolic phase, it is called the end-diastolic volume.

Contractility   Contractility is defined as an increased force of contraction *not* due to increased end-diastolic volume.

FACTORS THAT INFLUENCE STROKE VOLUME

End-diastolic Ventricular Volume

Starling's Heart-Lung Apparatus   The British physiologist Ernest Henry Starling (1866-1927) devised an apparatus for studying the responses of the heart to certain variables: temperature, plasma chemical concentrations, peripheral resistance, and venous pressure. Among other findings, Starling discovered that increasing the venous pressure stimulated the heart to increase its stroke volume. Increasing the venous pressure increases the rate at which blood returns to the heart (venous return) during diastole, which increases the end-diastolic volume. This automatic (intrinsic) response of the heart is directly related to the length of the cardiac muscle fibers at the end of diastole, and their length is determined by the end-diastolic volume (the degree to which the ventricles are distended).

Length-Tension Relationship   As cardiac muscle length increases, the tension generated during contraction increases. So, the more the ventricular muscle is stretched during the filling of the heart, the more forceful will be its response during contraction. The relationship between the end-diastolic volume (length of cardiac muscle fibers) and the force of contraction of the heart is known as *Starling's Law of the the Heart*.

Sympathetic Nerves

Contractility   Increased contractility is increased force of contraction; it is defined as an increased force of contraction *not* due to increased end-diastolic volume. Contractility is increased by the neurotransmitter norepinephrine (NE), which is released from the axon terminals of postganglionic sympathetic neurons. NE causes an increase in the movement of calcium ions into the cytosol of cardiac muscle cells; the increased calcium concentrations enhance the contraction mechanism, increasing the force of contraction.

Speed of Contraction and Relaxation   Norepinephrine also increases the rate of calcium transport back into the sarcoplasmic reticulum from the cytosol; this allows the muscle cells to relax, ending the contraction-relaxation sequence. Shortening the time needed for contraction-relaxation allows a greater fraction of the cardiac cycle to be available for passive filling.

Plasma Epinephrine

Like norepinephrine, epinephrine increases the stroke volume by increasing contractility.

STROKE VOLUME (SV)

Relationship Between End–diastolic Volume and SV

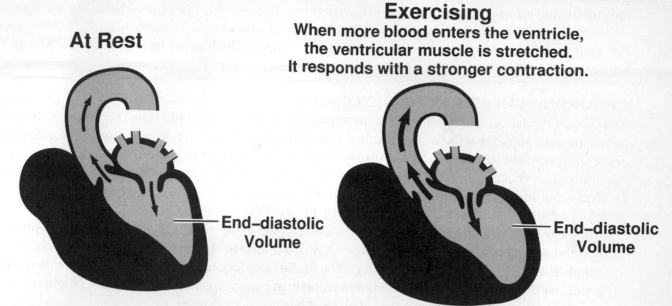

At Rest

Exercising
When more blood enters the ventricle,
the ventricular muscle is stretched.
It responds with a stronger contraction.

End–diastolic Volume

End–diastolic Volume

Hydraulic Pump Analogy

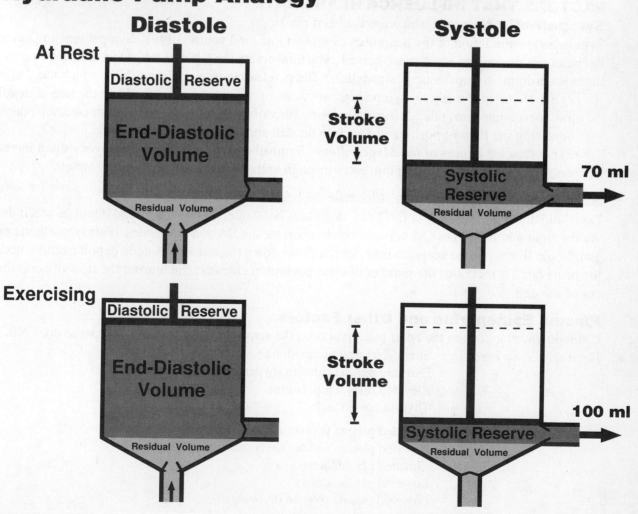

Diastole

Systole

At Rest

Diastolic Reserve

End-Diastolic Volume

Residual Volume

Stroke Volume

Systolic Reserve

Residual Volume

70 ml

Exercising

Diastolic Reserve

End-Diastolic Volume

Residual Volume

Stroke Volume

Systolic Reserve

Residual Volume

100 ml

HEART / Cardiac Output : Heart Rate

The heart rate is controlled primarily by balancing the inhibitory effects of parasympathetic nerves with the stimulating effects of sympathetic nerves. Rhythmic beating of the heart at a rate of approximately 100 beats per minute will occur in the complete absence of any nervous or hormonal influences. At rest, the major influence on heart rate is the parasympathetic input, which slows the rate to about 75 beats per minute.

CARDIOVASCULAR CENTER (CV Center)

The cardiovascular center consists of groups of neurons in the medulla oblongata (brain stem). It acts as an integrating center for reflexes that regulate heart rate, force of contraction, and blood vessel diameter. Some of its neurons stimulate the heart (cardio-accelerator center); some inhibit the heart (cardio-inhibitory center); and some cause the constriction of blood vessels (vasomotor center). The CV center receives input from higher brain regions, baroreceptors, and chemoreceptors. Both sympathetic and parasympathetic nerves leading to the heart originate in the CV center.

Baroreceptors Baroreceptors (pressoreceptors) located in the arch of the aorta and carotid sinuses (carotid arteries) monitor blood pressure. They detect changes in the blood pressure and relay the information to the cardiovascular center. The cardiovascular center integrates the information and sends out the appropriate impulses via sympathetic or parasympathetic nerve fibers. These responses regulate blood pressure as well as heart rate.

FACTORS THAT INFLUENCE HEART RATE

Sympathetic Nerves (increase the heart rate)

Sympathetic stimulation of the heart increases heart rate (and contractility). Sympathetic impulses reach the heart via the cardiac accelerator nerves, which innervate the SA and AV nodes and most portions of the myocardium. Sympathetic postganglionic fibers release norepinephrine (NE), which has 2 effects :

(1) SA Node (pacemaker) Sympathetic stimulation of the SA node speeds up the rate of depolarization, increasing heart rate. It increases the number of open sodium and calcium channels, thereby increasing the flow of positive charge into the cell and hastening depolarization.

(2) Contractile Fibers of the Myocardium Sympathetic stimulation of the myocardium increases contractility. It enhances calcium entry through voltage-gated slow calcium channels.

Parasympathetic Nerves (decrease the heart rate)

Parasympathetic stimulation of the heart decreases heart rate. Parasympathetic impulses reach the heart via the right and left vagus (X) nerves, which innervate the SA and AV nodes. Parasympathetic postganglionic fibers release acetylcholine, which slows down the rate of SA node depolarization, decreasing the heart rate. It increases the number of open potassium channels, increasing the flow of potassium ions out of the cell.

Plasma Epinephrine and Other Factors

Epinephrine : increases the heart rate. It acts on the same beta-adrenergic receptors as does NE.

Heart rate is *increased* by : Stress (physical or emotional).
Elevated plasma calcium (hypercalemia).
Elevated body temperatures.
Thyroid hormones.

Heart rate is *decreased* by : Elevated plasma potassium (hyperkalemia).
Elevated plasma sodium (hypernatremia).
Elevated pH (alkalosis).
Lowered pH (acidosis).
Lowered plasma oxygen (hypoxia).

HEART RATE: Sympathetic Control

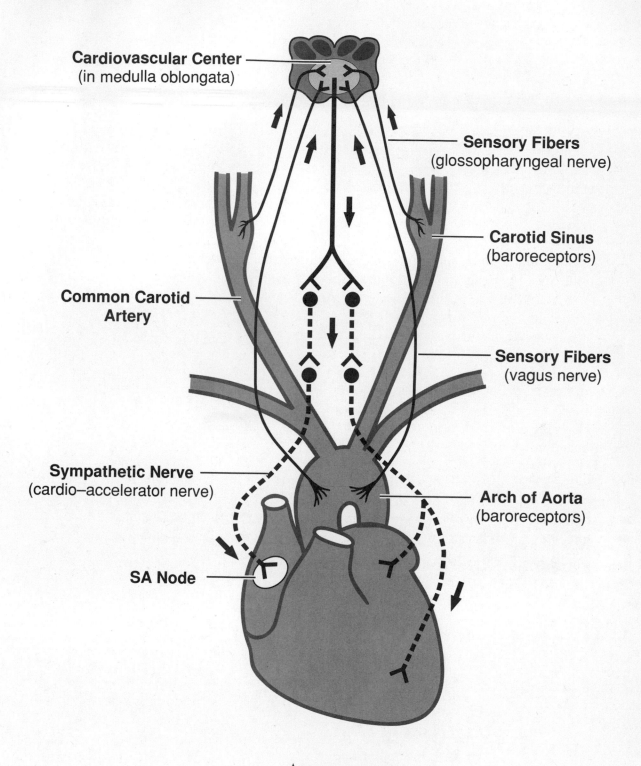

Cardiovascular Center
(in medulla oblongata)

Sensory Fibers
(glossopharyngeal nerve)

Carotid Sinus
(baroreceptors)

Common Carotid
Artery

Sensory Fibers
(vagus nerve)

Sympathetic Nerve
(cardio–accelerator nerve)

Arch of Aorta
(baroreceptors)

SA Node

↑ Heart Rate
(Norepinephrine released)

2 Blood Vessels

BLOOD VESSELS / Histology

All blood vessels, except capillaries, have three tissue layers: the inner layer is the tunica interna, the middle layer is the tunica media, and the outer layer is the tunica externa.
Lumen   The hollow center through which blood flows is called the lumen.

TISSUE LAYERS

Tunica Interna (inner coat)   Also called the tunica adventitia.
Endothelium   The inner coat (layer) of all blood vessels consists of endothelial cells (simple, squamous epithelium) that fit together like the parts of a jigsaw puzzle. These cells are in direct contact with the blood in the lumen. Some *collagen fibers* are present, which provide strength.
Basement Membrane   A basement membrane separates the tunica interna from the tunica media. (In arteries, a layer of elastic tissue called the *internal elastic lamina* is present; it is not present in veins.)

Tunica Media (middle coat)   The tunica media is usually the thickest coat.
Smooth Muscle Cells   The tunica media consists primarily of smooth muscle cells arranged in concentric layers around the tunica interna. *Gap junctions* between the smooth muscle cells facilitate the rapid transmission of electrical impulses (action potentials).
Elastin Fibers   Elastin (elastic) fibers are interspersed among the smooth muscle cells, giving elasticity to the vessel walls.

Tunica Externa (outer coat)
Collagen and Elastin Fibers   The tunica adventitia consists primarily of longitudinally oriented collagen and elastin fibers. In arteries, a layer of elastic tissue called the *external elastic lamina* separates the tunica externa from the tunica media.

> *Vasa vasorum* (vessels of the vessel)   Vasa vasorum are capillaries that penetrate the tunica externa in large arteries and veins. They are especially prevalent in large veins, since the blood in the lumens is low in oxygen and nutrients, making it difficult for sufficient materials to diffuse from the blood in the lumens of the veins to the cells deep in the tunica externa.
>
> *Sympathetic Nerves*   Sympathetic nerves have axon terminals in the tunica externa that release norepinephrine, which must diffuse several micrometers to the smooth muscle cells in the tunica media. Sympathetic input regulates the degree of muscle contraction and, therefore, the diameter of the vessel lumen.
>
> *Sensory Nerve Endings*   Sensory nerve endings are present in the walls of some arteries. Stretch receptors in the walls of the carotid sinus and arch of the aorta monitor blood pressure; chemoreceptors in the walls of carotid and aortic bodies monitor gas concentrations.

TYPES OF BLOOD VESSELS

In the systemic circulatory system arteries and arterioles carry blood with nutrients and oxygen to the tissues; the exchange of nutrients, gases, and metabolic waste products between blood and tissue cells occurs in the capillaries; venules and veins carry blood back to the heart. The structure of each type of vessel reflects its function.

> *Arteries*   Carry blood away from the heart toward organs.
> *Arterioles*   Small vessels that carry blood from arteries to capillaries.
> *Capillaries*   Microscopic vessels that connect arterioles to venules.
> *Venules*   Small vessels that drain blood from capillaries into veins.
> *Veins*   Carry blood from venules to the heart.

BLOOD VESSEL WALLS

All blood vessel walls (except capillaries)
are composed of three basic tissue layers

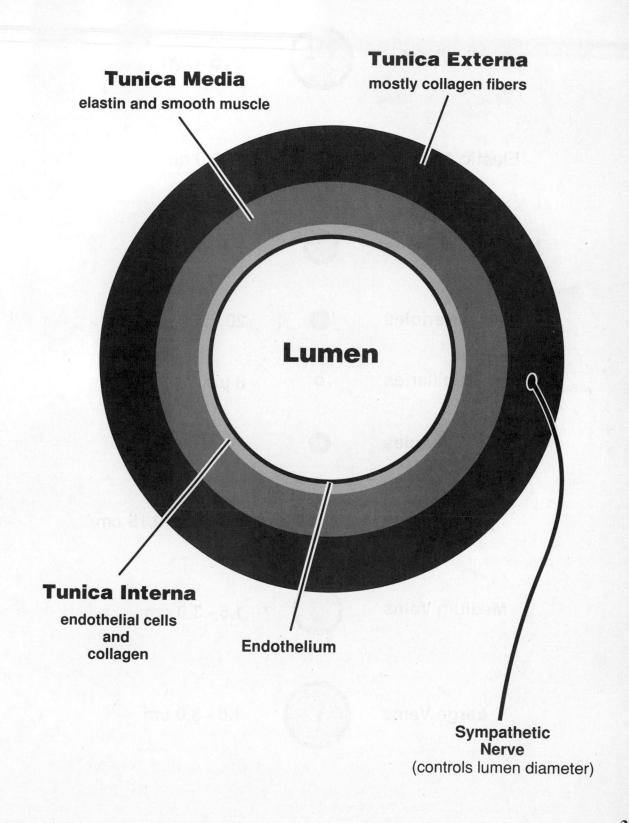

Tunica Media
elastin and smooth muscle

Tunica Externa
mostly collagen fibers

Lumen

Tunica Interna
endothelial cells
and
collagen

Endothelium

**Sympathetic
Nerve**
(controls lumen diameter)

BLOOD VESSEL DIAMETERS
Lumen Diameters

Aorta	← →	**2.5 cm**
Elastic Arteries		1 - 2.0 cm
Muscular Arteries		0.1 - 1.0 cm
Arterioles		20 - 200 μm
Capillaries		8 μm
Venules		20 - 500 μm
Small Veins		0.5 mm - 0.15 cm
Medium Veins		1.5 - 3.0 cm
Large Veins		1.5 - 3.0 cm

BLOOD VESSEL WALL COMPOSITION

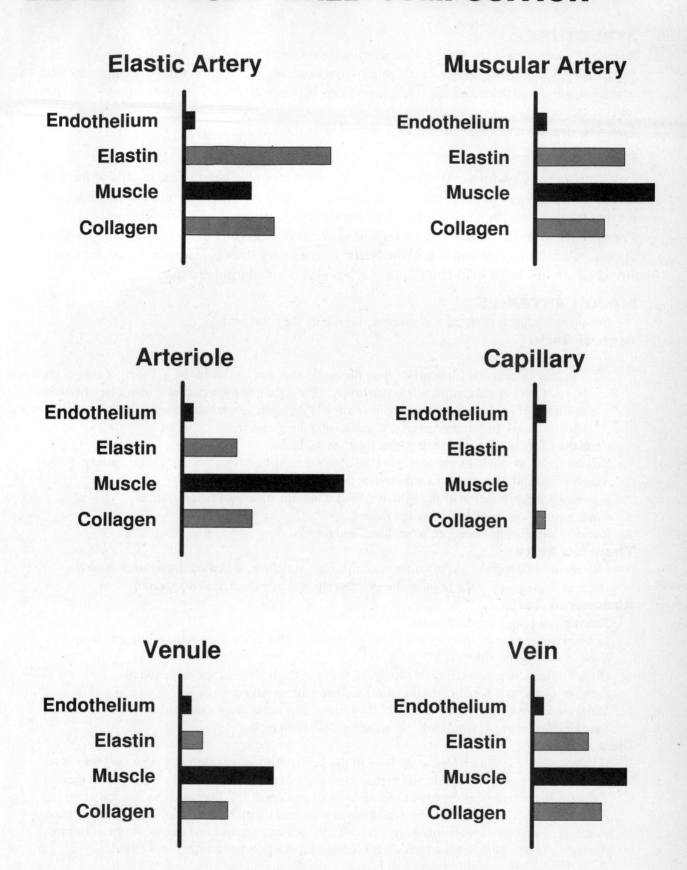

BLOOD VESSELS / Arteries

STRUCTURE
Elastic (Conducting) Arteries   Large arteries are referred to as elastic arteries.
Muscular (Distributing) Arteries   Medium-sized arteries are referred to as muscular arteries.
Anastomoses   Anastomoses are interconnections between arteries that allow for alternate pathways of blood flow.
End Arteries   Arteries that do not anastomose are called end arteries.

FUNCTIONS
Low-Resistance Conduits   Arteries carry blood away from the heart to the organs of the body. Because they have relatively large lumens, they offer little resistance to blood flow. For this reason, the pressure remains relatively constant as blood passes through the arteries.
Pressure Reservoirs   Arteries also function as pressure reservoirs or secondary pumps. During systole, when blood is pumped into the elastic arteries they stretch. The elastic recoil of the stretched arteries helps maintain the arterial blood pressure during diastole.

MAJOR ARTERIES
Coronary : branch from the ascending aorta; supply the heart muscle.
Arch of Aorta
Brachiocephalic Trunk
> The brachiocephalic trunk arises from the aortic arch and carries blood to the right side of the upper body; it becomes the right subclavian artery. The right common carotid artery arises from the junction between the brachiocephalic trunk and the right subclavian artery. The left subclavian and left common carotid arteries arise directly from the aortic arch.

Common Carotid : the main artery that supplies the brain.
Subclavian :   the main artery supplying the upper extremities; becomes the axillary artery.
Axillary : a continuation of the subclavian; becomes the brachial artery.
Brachial : a continuation of the axillary; divides into the ulnar and radial arteries.
Ulnar : supplies the elbow joint and forearm.
Radial : supplies the forearm, wrist, hand, and fingers.
Thoracic Aorta
Intercostals (10 pairs) : supply intercostal muscles, vertebrae, spinal cord, and back muscles.
Other branches supply the bronchi, lungs, esophagus, percardium, and diaphragm.
Abdominal Aorta
Phrenic : supplies the diaphragm.
Celiac Trunk (gastric, splenic, and hepatic arteries) : supply the stomach, spleen, and liver.
Renal : supply the kidneys.
Gonadal (testicular or ovarian) : supply the testes in the male, ovaries in the female.
Lumbar (4 pairs) : supply the abdominal wall and the spinal cord.
Superior Mesenteric : supplies the small intestine, appendix, and ascending and transverse colon.
Inferior Mesenteric : supplies the descending colon and rectum.
Iliac Arteries
Common Iliac : aorta divides at the level of the pelvic brim into the left and right common iliac.
Internal Iliac : supplies pelvic and gluteal muscles, external genitalia, and visceral structures.
External Iliac : supplies the lower abdominal wall and upper leg; becomes the femoral artery.
Femoral : supplies the groin, lower abdominal wall, and thigh; becomes popliteal artery at knee.
Popliteal : supplies knee joint, thigh, and calf; divides into anterior and posterior tibial arteries.
Anterior Tibial : supplies the lower leg; becomes the dorsalis pedis artery in the foot.
Posterior Tibial : supplies lower leg; becomes plantar arch in the foot.
Peroneal : a branch of the posterior tibial artery; supplies the lower leg.

MAJOR ARTERIES

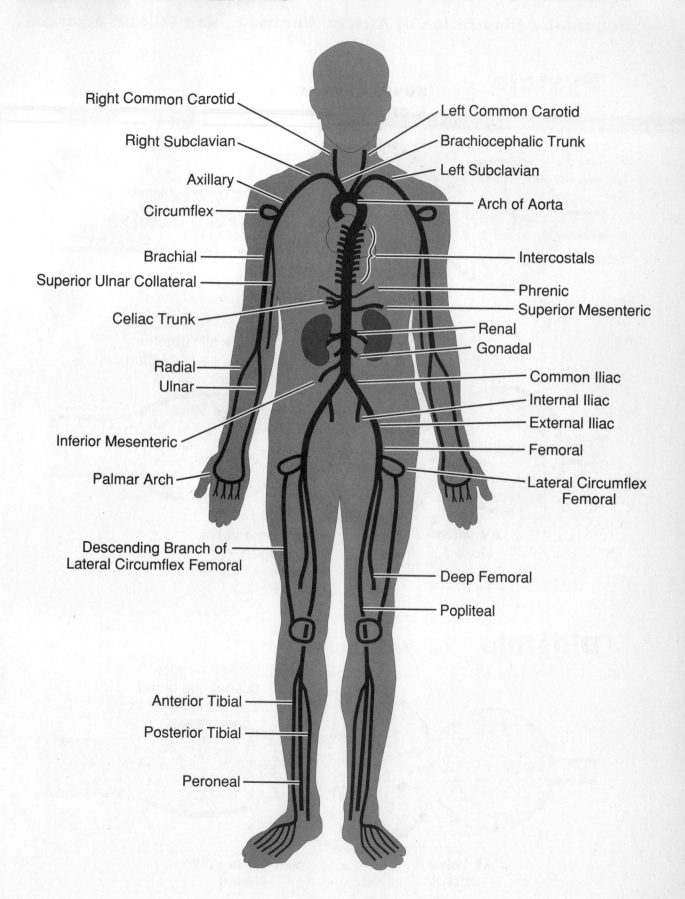

Right Common Carotid

Right Subclavian

Axillary

Circumflex

Brachial

Superior Ulnar Collateral

Celiac Trunk

Radial

Ulnar

Inferior Mesenteric

Palmar Arch

Descending Branch of
Lateral Circumflex Femoral

Anterior Tibial

Posterior Tibial

Peroneal

Left Common Carotid

Brachiocephalic Trunk

Left Subclavian

Arch of Aorta

Intercostals

Phrenic

Superior Mesenteric

Renal

Gonadal

Common Iliac

Internal Iliac

External Iliac

Femoral

Lateral Circumflex
Femoral

Deep Femoral

Popliteal

ELASTIC ARTERIES : Elastic Recoil
Schematic Illustration of Atrium, Ventricle, and Elastic Arteries

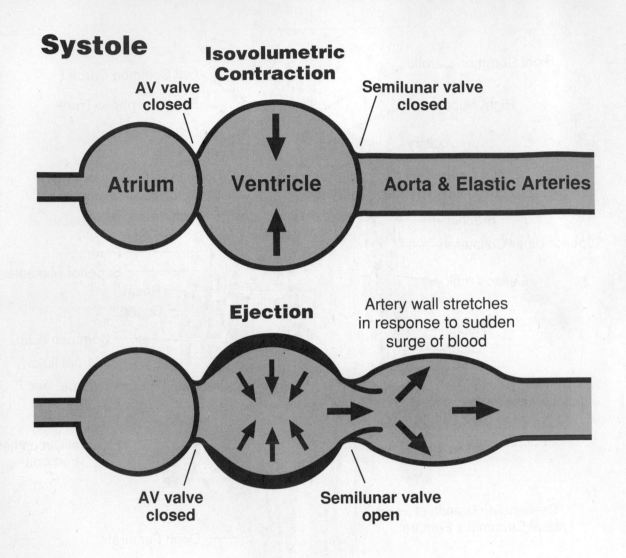

Systole

Isovolumetric Contraction

AV valve closed

Semilunar valve closed

Atrium

Ventricle

Aorta & Elastic Arteries

Ejection

Artery wall stretches in response to sudden surge of blood

AV valve closed

Semilunar valve open

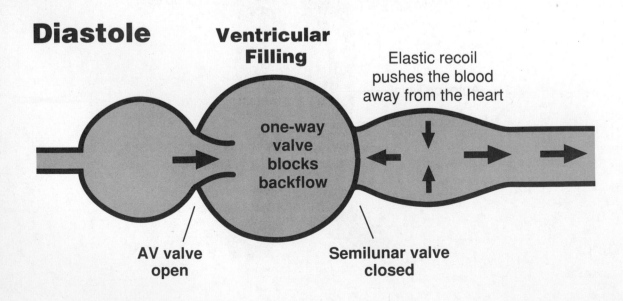

Diastole

Ventricular Filling

Elastic recoil pushes the blood away from the heart

one-way valve blocks backflow

AV valve open

Semilunar valve closed

ATHEROSCLEROSIS

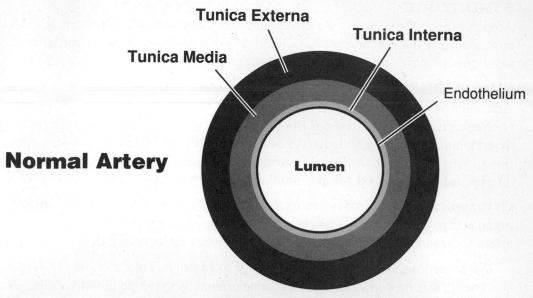

Tunica Externa

Tunica Interna

Tunica Media

Endothelium

Normal Artery

Lumen

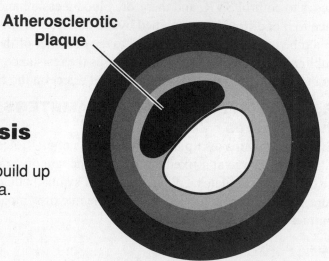

Atherosclerotic
Plaque

Moderate
Atherosclerosis

Fatty deposits begin to build up
in the tunica interna.

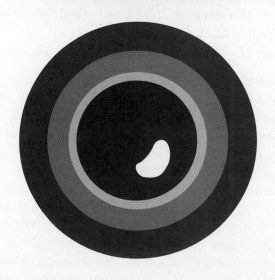

Extreme
Atherosclerosis

Fatty deposits
and calcium buildup;
blockage almost total.

BLOOD VESSELS / Arterioles

STRUCTURE
Arteriole means little artery. Arterioles are small, almost microscopic arteries that carry blood from muscular (distributing) arteries to capillaries. As arterioles approach capillaries their walls become more muscular and less elastic in composition.

FUNCTIONS
Arterioles have two main functions :

(1) Regulation of Mean Arterial Pressure   When arterioles throughout the body constrict in response to stimulation by sympathetic nerves or hormones, the arterial blood pressure rises. The vasoconstriction of arterioles slows the blood flow into the capillary beds, and this causes blood to back up in the arteries, raising the blood volume and therefore the blood pressure.

(2) Control of Blood Distribution to the Various Organs   The volume of blood flow to a particular organ is regulated by the diameters of the arterioles leading to that organ. When exercising, the arterioles leading to skeletal muscles dilate, allowing an increased flow of blood to the muscles.

> *Systemic Vascular Resistance* (SVR) *(also known as Total Peripheral Resistance or TPR)* The SVR is the total vascular resistance offered by systemic blood vessels. A major function of arterioles is to control SVR, and therefore blood pressure and blood flow to particular organs. The resistance to blood flow is determined by the diameter of the arterioles. The flow of any liquid through a tube is inversely proportional to the diameter of the tube to the 4th power. This means that doubling the diameter of a tube decreases the resistance 16-fold. Thus, a very small change in the diameter of an arteriole has a very marked effect on the flow of blood.

FACTORS THAT AFFECT LUMEN DIAMETERS
Sympathetic Nerves
The smooth muscle that makes up the tunica externa of arterioles is innervated by sympathetic nerves which constantly discharge at a fixed basal rate. The rate of sympathetic discharge determines whether the arteriole constricts or dilates. When the rate of sympathetic discharge is increased, the muscles contract more, causing vasoconstriction; when the rate of sympathetic discharge is decreased, the muscles contract less, causing vasodilation.

Hormones
Epinephrine   Epinephrine causes general vasoconstriction of arterioles, raising the blood pressure.

Antidiuretic Hormone (ADH)   (also called *Vasopressin*) Antidiuretic hormone causes general vasoconstriction of blood vessels.

Angiotensin II   Angiotensin II also causes general vasoconstriction of blood vessels.

Local Controls (Autoregulation)
Metabolic Activity (active hyperemia) When cells of a given organ become more active, as in the case of skeletal muscles during physical exercise, the result is *decreased* concentrations of oxygen in the surrounding ECF and *increased* concentrations of carbon dioxide, hydrogen ions, potassium ions, adenosine, prostaglandins, and bradykinins. These changes in the chemical concentrations of ECF stimulate *arteriolar vasodilation*, increasing the flow of blood to the region.

Reduced Blood Pressure   When arterial blood pressure is reduced there is a decreased blood flow to all organs. The oxygen supply is reduced and metabolic wastes accumulate in the ECF. These changes have the same effect as increased metabolic activity: arteriolar vasodilation.

Injury or Infection (inflammatory response) Tissue damage causes the release of vasodilator chemicals such as histamine and kinins. Vasodilation of local arterioles facilitates the transport of white blood cells and plasma proteins (complement and antibodies) to the infected area.

ARTERIOLE

The lumen diameter of arterioles regulates the distribution of blood and helps maintain the normal arterial blood pressure.

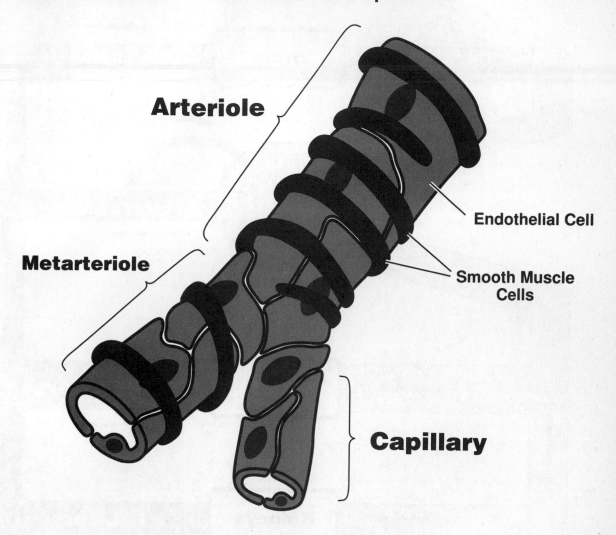

Arteriole

Endothelial Cell

Smooth Muscle Cells

Metarteriole

Capillary

Lumen Diameter

The lumen diameter is inversely proportional to the frequency of sympathetic nerve impulses.

Diameter Range : 20 - 200 μm

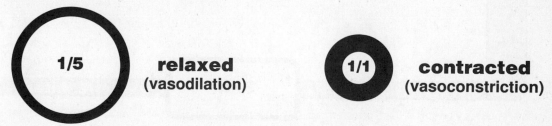

1/5 relaxed (vasodilation)

1/1 contracted (vasoconstriction)

ARTERIOLES : Distribution of Blood

The lumen diameters of the arterioles leading to an organ determine the volume of blood flow to that organ.

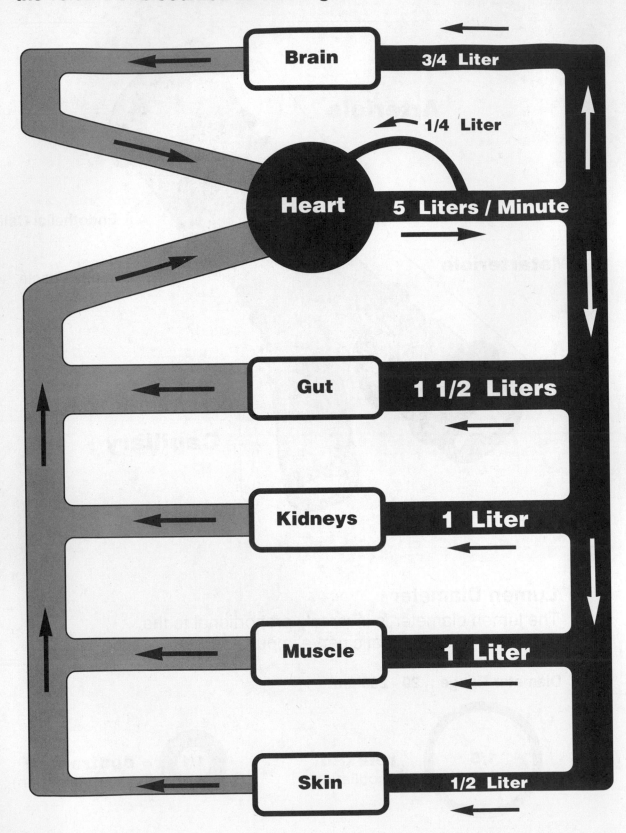

ARTERIOLES : Distribution of Blood to the Skin

Blood flow to the skin is regulated by the lumen diameters of the arterioles carrying blood to the skin.

The degree of vasoconstriction of the arterioles is directly proportional to the degree of stimulation by sympathetic nerves.

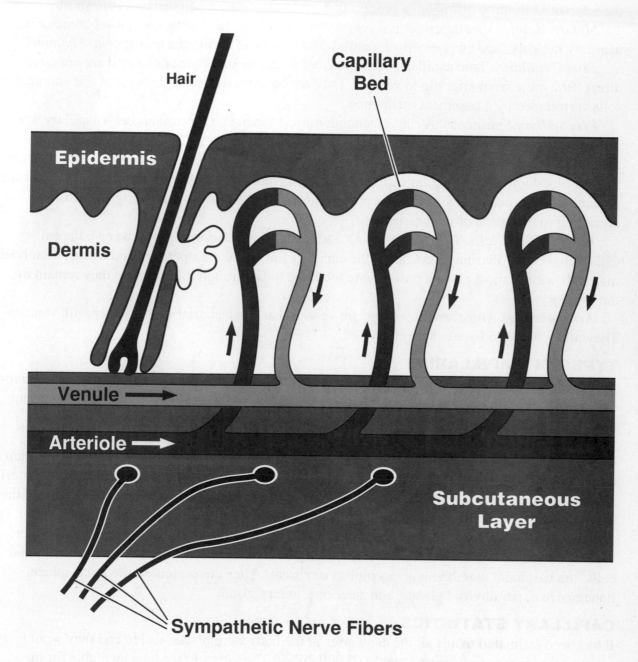

BLOOD VESSELS / Capillaries : Microcirculation

STRUCTURE

Capillary Bed A capillary bed is a network of microscopic blood vessels where exchange of materials occurs between the blood and tissue cells. Every tissue cell is usually within two or three cell diameters from a capillary. The proximity is important, since materials travel through the interstitial fluid by diffusion, a process that is efficient only when distances are short.

Metarterioles A metarteriole is a vessel that emerges from an arteriole, passes through the capillary network, and empties into a venule. The distal end is called a *thoroughfare channel*.

True Capillary True capillaries emerge from arterioles or metarterioles and are not on the direct flow route from arteriole to venule. They are composed of a single layer of flat endothelial cells surrounded by a basement membrane.

Precapillary Sphincter A ring of smooth muscle (sphincter) surrounds each capillary where it branches from an arteriole. High oxygen concentrations in the ECF, which indicate low metabolic activity in nearby tissue cells, causes a precapillary sphincter to contract, stopping the flow of blood into that particular capillary. At any given moment, only a small percentage of the precapillary sphincters in the body are open. They are self-regulating, opening and closing according to the needs of the nearby cells.

Intercellular Clefts (Capillary Pores) Intercellular clefts are spaces between adjacent endothelial cells. Plasma filters out of the capillary through these openings and carries dissolved materials with it; most plasma proteins are too large to fit through the pores, so they remain in the capillary.

Arteriovenous Anastomosis These are vessels that connect arterioles directly with venules. They allow blood to bypass a capillary bed.

TYPES OF CAPILLARIES

Continuous Capillary Except for the intercellular clefts, the plasma membranes of continuous capillaries form a continuous, uninterrupted ring around the capillary. They are present in the lungs, smooth muscle, skeletal muscle, and connective tissue.

Fenestrated Capillary In some capillaries the endothelial cells appear to be perforated. These fenestrations (little windows) are about 70 nm in diameter and are closed by a diaphragm that is thinner than the cell membrane. These openings allow for more rapid exchange of materials between the blood and the tissues. They are present in kidneys, endocrine glands, villi of the small intestine, ciliary processes of the eye, and the choroid plexuses of the brain.

Sinusoidal Capillary (Sinusoids) Sinusoidal capillaries have larger diameters than other capillaries and have a more irregular shape. They contain wide spaces between the endothelial cells; the basement membrane is incomplete or absent. They are present in the liver, spleen, bone marrow, parathyroid glands, and anterior pituitary gland.

CAPILLARY STATISTICS

It has been estimated that if all the capillaries in the body were placed end to end they would stretch for a distance of approximately 60,000 miles. The total surface area available for the exchange of materials is about 6000 square meters. The total cross-sectional area of all the capillaries combined is about 5000 cm^2 (the cross-sectional area of the aorta is only $3 - 5$ cm^2). The average capillary is about 1 mm long and has a lumen diameter of about 8 micrometers; because of the small diameter, red blood cells must pass through one at a time. The velocity of blood flow in a capillary is less than 0.1 cm/sec. The concentration of capillaries in a given tissue is directly proportional to the metabolic activity of the cells.

CAPILLARY BED

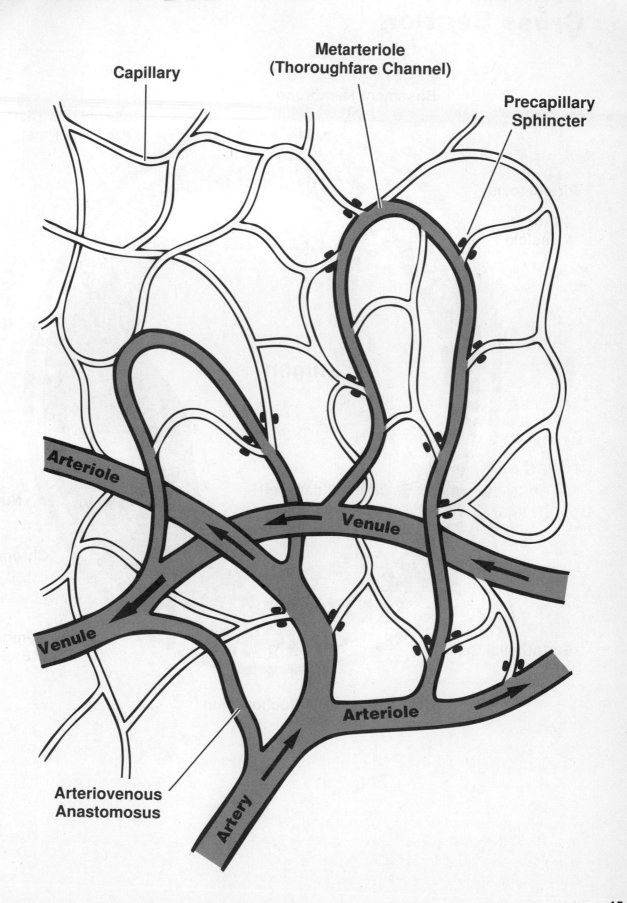

Capillary

Metarteriole
(Thoroughfare Channel)

Precapillary
Sphincter

Arteriole

Venule

Venule

Arteriole

Arteriovenous
Anastomosus

Artery

CAPILLARY
Cross Section

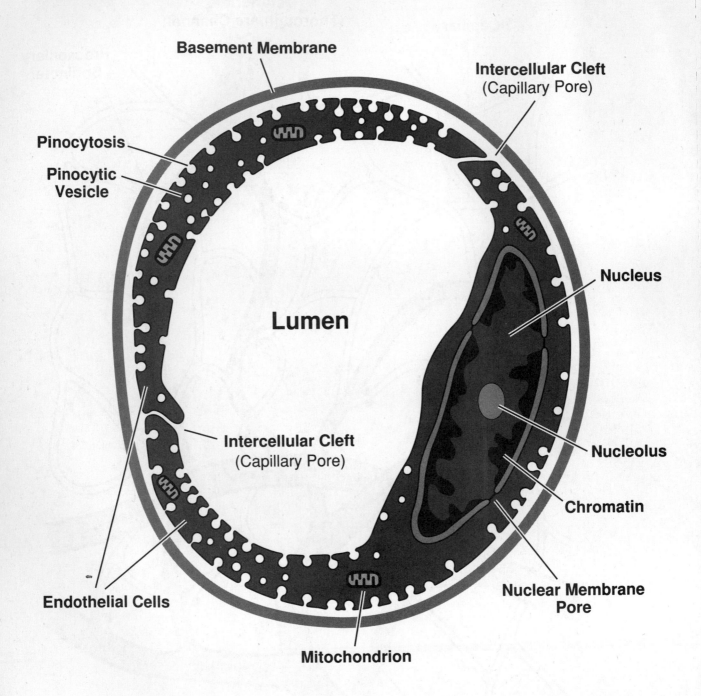

Basement Membrane

Intercellular Cleft
(Capillary Pore)

Pinocytosis

Pinocytic
Vesicle

Nucleus

Lumen

Intercellular Cleft
(Capillary Pore)

Nucleolus

Chromatin

Nuclear Membrane
Pore

Endothelial Cells

Mitochondrion

TYPES OF CAPILLARIES

Continuous Capillary

found in :
    lungs
    smooth muscle
    skeletal muscle
    connective tissues

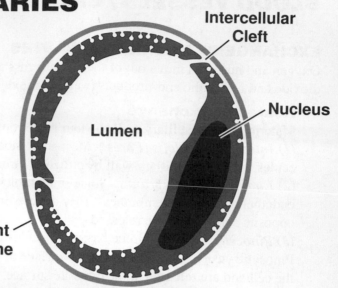

Intercellular Cleft

Nucleus

Lumen

Basement Membrane

Fenestrated Capillary

found in :
    kidneys
    endocrine glands
    villi of small intestine
    ciliary processes of the eye
    choroid plexuses of the brain

Basement Membrane

Intercellular Cleft

Lumen

Fenestrations

Sinusoidal Capillary

found in :
    liver
    spleen
    bone marrow
    parathyroid glands
    anterior pituitary gland

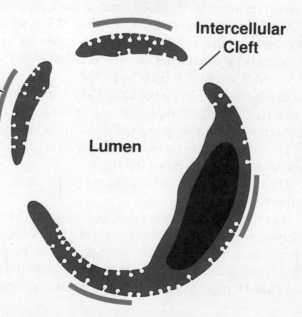

Intercellular Cleft

Basement Membrane

Lumen

BLOOD VESSELS / Capillaries : Exchange of Materials

EXCHANGE OF NUTRIENTS, WASTES, AND GASES
Oxygen and nutrients move out of the blood across the capillary wall into the interstitial fluid; carbon dioxide and metabolic end-products (wastes) move in the opposite direction.

Routes of Exchange
Materials cross capillary walls by four basic routes :

(1) Intercellular Clefts (Pores) Most substances, including water and small hydrophilic molecules, cross the capillary wall by diffusion through the endothelial junctions (pores).

(2) Endothelial Membranes Some small molecules can diffuse or be actively transported across endothelial plasma membranes. They diffuse through the cytoplasm of the endothelial cell to the opposite surface and are released.

(3) Pinocytic Vesicles Some larger molecules pass through the endothelial cells by pinocytosis. Pinocytic vesicles are formed on one surface of the cell; they diffuse through the cytoplasm of the cell and are released at the opposite surface.

(4) Fenestrations (little windows) When capillaries are perforated with fenestrations, large molecules can pass quickly through the fenestrations by diffusion.

Mechanisms for Exchange
Materials pass through capillary walls by three basic mechanisms :

(1) Diffusion Diffusion is the movement of molecules or ions from a region of higher concentration to one of lower concentration until equilibrium is reached. It is a passive process.

(2) Vesicular Transport (endocytosis and exocytosis) Endocytosis includes phagocytosis ("cell eating") and pinocytosis ("cell drinking"). In exocytosis secretory vesicles fuse with the plasma membrane and release their contents into the ECF (plasma or interstitial fluid).

(3) Bulk Flow (filtration and absorption) Bulk flow is the movement of a fluid (liquid or gas) from a region of higher pressure to one of lower pressure. It is a passive process.

FLUID EXCHANGE
Hydrostatic and Osmotic Pressures As blood flows through a capillary, the blood hydrostatic pressure (BHP) tends to push fluid out through the capillary pores. The blood colloid osmotic pressure (BCOP), which is caused by the difference in water concentrations in the plasma and interstitial fluid, tends to pull water from the interstitial fluid into the capillary. There is a very small interstitial fluid osmotic pressure (IFOP) which tends to move fluid out of the capillaries into the interstitial fluid.

Net Filtration Pressure (NFP) The NFP is used to show the direction of fluid movement. Whether fluids leave or enter capillaries depends on how the hydrostatic and osmotic pressures relate to each other. The formula for calculating the NFP is the following :

$$NFP = (BHP + IFOP) - BCOP$$

The BHP at the arterial end of a capillary is about 35 mm Hg; at the venous end it has dropped to about 16 mm Hg. The BCOP pulling water into both ends of the capillary is approximately 26 mm Hg. The IFOP is about 1 mm Hg along the length of the capillary.

The net force at the arterial end is equal to (35 + 1) − 26 = 10 mm Hg, forcing plasma out of the capillary by a process called filtration.

The net force at the venous end is equal to (16 + 1) − 26 = −9 mm Hg, pulling water back into the capillary by osmosis.

As a result of this fluid exchange, a constant flow of interstitial fluid washes over the tissue cells, supplying oxygen and nutrients, and carrying away carbon dioxide and metabolic end-products (wastes). This mechanism is not perfect, since more fluid leaves the capillary than re-enters. Another set of tubes called lymphatic capillaries drain the excess interstitial fluid from the tissue spaces and return the fluid (now called lymph) to the blood via lymphatic vessels, which empty into large veins near the heart.

CAPILLARY : Exchange of Food and Waste

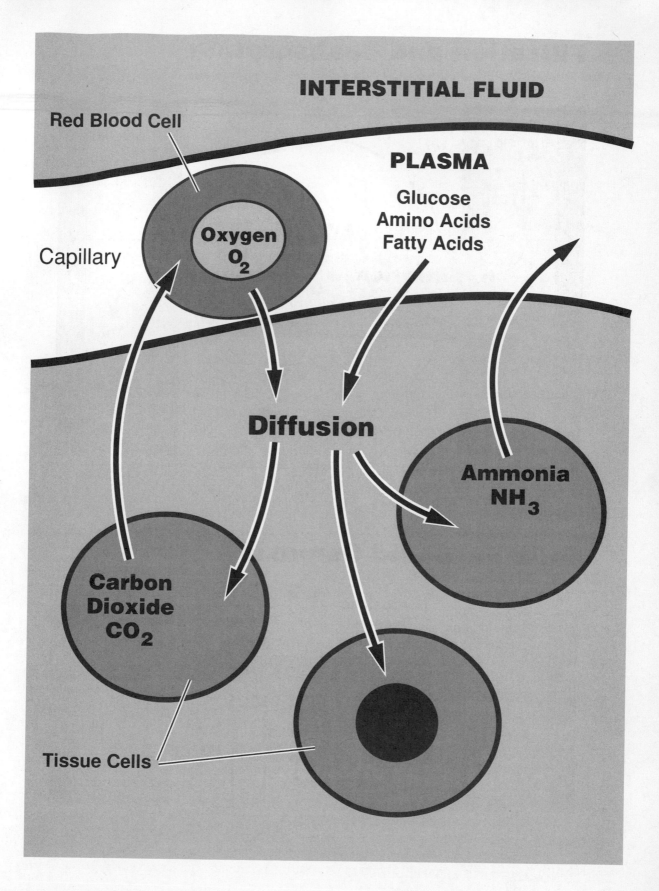

CAPILLARY : Exchange of Fluid

Filtration and Reabsorption

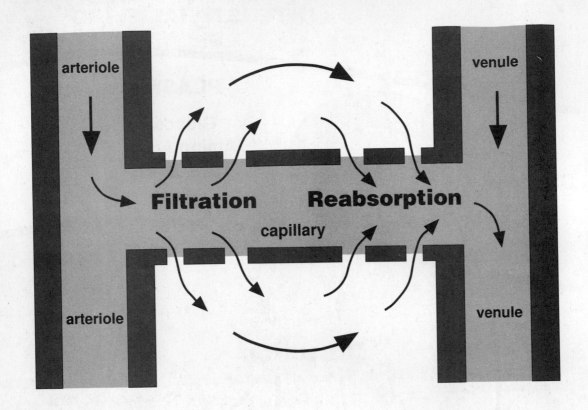

Bulk Flow and Osmosis

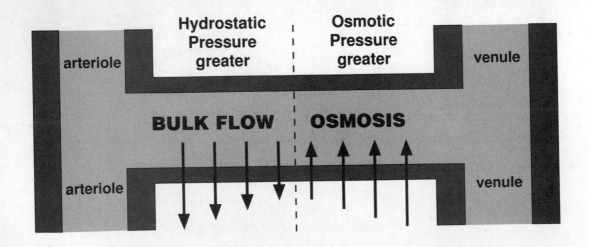

CAPILLARY: Pressure Gradients

Numbers : the pressure in mm Hg.
Arrows : the direction that fluid moves.

BHP : Blood Hydrostatic Pressure
IFOP : Interstitial Fluid Osmotic Pressure
BCOP : Blood Colloid Osmotic Pressure

Hydrostatic Pressures

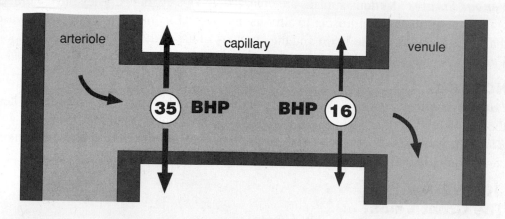

Osmotic Pressures (average values)

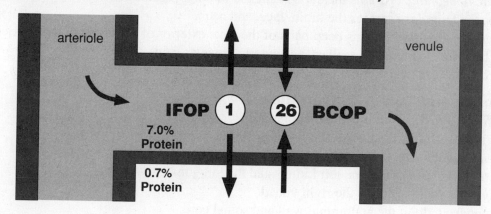

Net Pressures = BHP + IFOP – BCOP

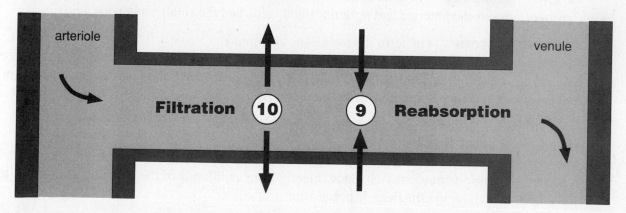

BLOOD VESSELS / Veins

STRUCTURE

Tissue Layers   Compared to arteries, veins have a thinner tunica interna and media; they have a thicker tunica externa.

Valves   Veins contain one-way valves to prevent the backflow of blood.

Venous Sinuses   Venous sinuses are enlarged venous channels. They have a thin endothelial wall that has no smooth muscle to alter its diameter. Examples are intracranial vascular sinuses that drain blood from the brain and the coronary sinus of the heart.

Venules   Venules are small vessels that drain blood from capillaries to veins.

FUNCTIONS

Low-Resistance Conduits   Veins carry deoxygenated blood from organs to the heart. Because they have relatively large lumens, they offer little resistance to blood flow.

Blood Reservoirs   At rest, systemic veins contain about 60% of the blood volume. This blood can be quickly diverted to other vessels if the need arises.

MAJOR VEINS

The Great Veins

Superior Vena Cava : drains the head and upper extremities.

Inferior Vena Cava : drains the torso and lower extremities.

Head and Upper Extremities

Brachiocephalic : drains the subclavian and internal jugular veins.

Internal Jugular : drains the brain, face, and neck.

External Jugular : drains deep parts of the face, exterior of the cranium, and auricular veins.

Subclavian : drains the axillary and external jugular veins.

Axillary : drains the upper extremity (the brachial, cephalic, and basilic veins)

Torso and Lower Extremities

Inferior Phrenic : drains the diaphragm.

Hepatic : drains the liver.

Renal : drains the kidney.

Left Gonadal : drains the left kidney and the left gonad.

Right Gonadal : drains the right gonad.

Lumbars : drain the abdominal wall and spinal cord.

Common Iliac : drains the lower extremity and pelvic region.

Internal Iliac : drains gluteal and thigh muscles, urinary bladder, rectum, and reproductive organs.

External Iliac : drains the femoral and great saphenous veins.

Femoral : drains deep structures of the thigh.

Popliteal : drains the anterior and posterior tibial veins and the small saphenous vein.

Azygos System   (The term *azygos* means unpaired.)

Most structures of the thorax (chest) are drained by a network of veins called the azygos system. The azygos system drains blood from the lungs, esophagus, pericardium, vertebrae, diaphragm, and thoracic spinal cord. It connects with the superior vena cava and the tributaries of the inferior vena cava.

Hepatic Portal System

The hepatic portal system drains blood from the pancreas, spleen, stomach, intestine, and gallbladder. It transports nutrient-rich blood directly from capillaries of the gastrointestinal tract to sinusoids of the liver via the hepatic portal vein.

MAJOR VEINS

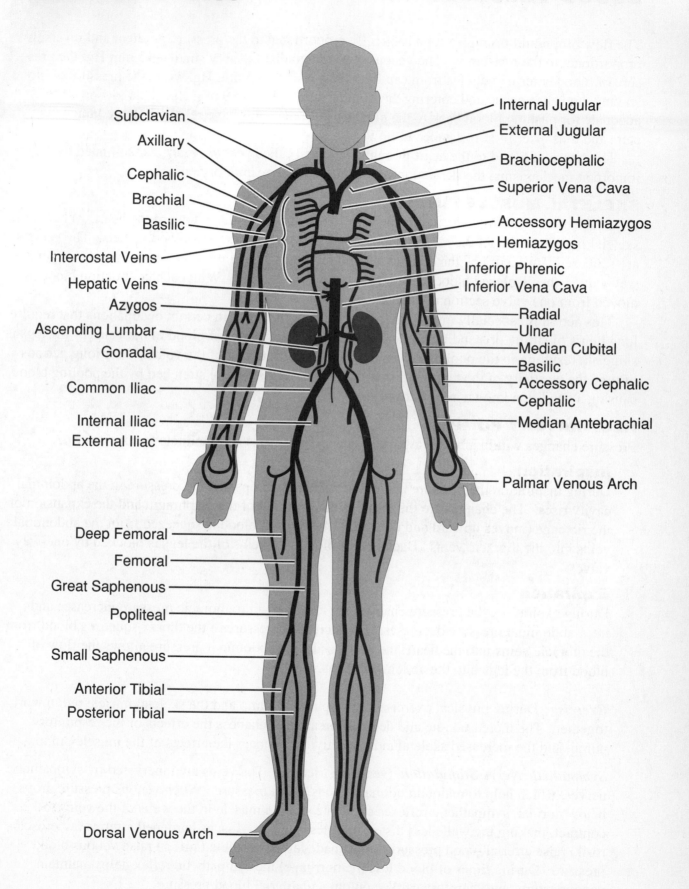

Subclavian
Axillary
Cephalic
Brachial
Basilic
Intercostal Veins
Hepatic Veins
Azygos
Ascending Lumbar
Gonadal
Common Iliac
Internal Iliac
External Iliac

Deep Femoral
Femoral
Great Saphenous
Popliteal
Small Saphenous
Anterior Tibial
Posterior Tibial

Dorsal Venous Arch

Internal Jugular
External Jugular
Brachiocephalic
Superior Vena Cava
Accessory Hemiazygos
Hemiazygos
Inferior Phrenic
Inferior Vena Cava
Radial
Ulnar
Median Cubital
Basilic
Accessory Cephalic
Cephalic
Median Antebrachial

Palmar Venous Arch

BLOOD VESSELS / Veins : Venous Return

The flow of a liquid through a tube is directly proportional to the pressure gradient and inversely proportional to the resistance. The venous pressure gradient is very small—15 mm Hg; the pressure of blood entering venules from capillary beds is about 15 mm Hg, while the pressure of blood leaving the venae cavae and entering the right atrium is close to 0 mm Hg. This low pressure is adequate for pushing blood back to the heart because the veins have relatively large lumen diameters and thus offer little resistance to flow.

The return of blood to the heart through the veins, called *venous return*, is facilitated by two important mechanisms: the skeletal muscle pump and the respiratory pump.

SKELETAL MUSCLE PUMP

Physical exercise and movement in general help squeeze blood back toward the heart. When skeletal muscles contract they thicken and bulge, pressing on adjacent blood vessels. The vessels are squeezed ("milked") by the contracting and relaxing skeletal muscles. Since veins contain one-way valves, the displaced blood always moves toward the heart. With each contraction blood is moved from one valve section to another.

This action is especially important for the veins of the legs. In certain occupations that require long hours of sitting or standing without walking, the movement of blood in the veins of the legs is sluggish, resulting in the pooling of venous blood and stretching of the veins. Over long periods of time the elasticity of the veins is decreased and the veins remain stretched by the pooling blood, causing a condition known as *varicose veins*.

RESPIRATORY PUMP

Pressure changes within a body cavity also squeeze the veins and facilitate venous return.

Inspiration

During inspiration the pressure in the thoracic cavity drops and the pressure in the abdominal cavity rises. The changes are the result of the lowering of the diaphragm and the expansion of the rib cage (moves upward and outward). As a result, blood is squeezed from the abdominal veins into the thoracic veins. Backflow of blood into veins of the legs is blocked by one-way valves.

Expiration

During expiration, the pressure changes are reversed—intrathoracic pressure increases and intra-abdominal pressure decreases. The increased pressure in the thorax squeezes blood from the thoracic veins into the heart; the decreased intra-abdominal pressure allows the flow of blood from the legs into the abdominal veins.

Exercise During physical exercise, the respiratory pump and the skeletal muscle pump work together. The increased rate and depth of breathing enhances the effects of the respiratory pump, and the increased skeletal muscle activity enhances the effects of the muscle pump.

Sympathetic Nerve Stimulation (venoconstriction) The veins are innervated by sympathetic nerves, which help to maintain normal venous blood pressure. When venous pressure drops below normal, sympathetic reflexes stimulate smooth muscle in the walls of the veins to contract, making the walls less distensible (less elastic). Just as hardened arteries (atherosclerosis) raise arterial blood pressure, veins made less distensible (stiffer) raise venous blood pressure. During times of blood loss (hemorrhage) the sympathetic reflex helps maintain venous return, and therefore cardiac output and arterial blood pressure.

VENOUS RETURN
Body Cavities

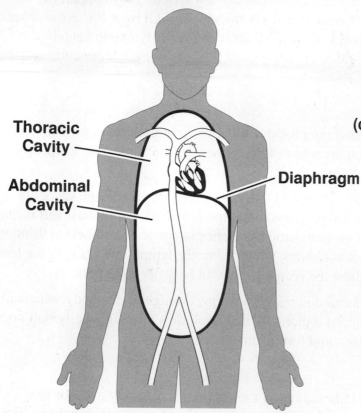

Thoracic Cavity

Abdominal Cavity

Diaphragm

Muscle Pump

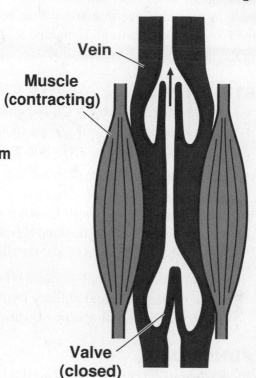

Vein

Muscle (contracting)

Valve (closed)

Respiratory Pump

Inspiration
↑ flow into thoracic veins

↓ intrathoracic pressure

↑ intra-abdominal pressure

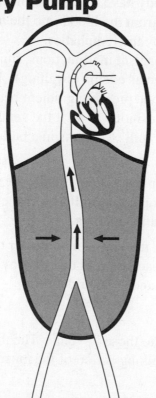

Expiration
↑ flow into abdominal veins

↑ intrathoracic pressure

↓ intra-abdominal pressure

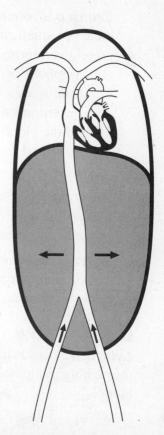

BLOOD VESSELS / Lymphatic Vessels

Technically, the lymphatic vessels are not part of the circulatory system; they are part of the immune system. They are a system of vessels that carry interstitial fluid from the tissue spaces back to the veins; the interstitial fluid is called lymph after it enters the lymphatic capillaries. As the lymph passes through lymph nodes microorganisms are filtered out by lymphocytes residing in the nodes.

STRUCTURES

Lymphatic Capillaries   Closed-ended lymphatic capillaries are present in almost all organs of the body. These thin-walled capillaries have large pores and are permeable to all interstitial fluid constituents, including protein.

Lymph and Lymphatic Vessels   *Blood plasma* that has filtered into the tissue spaces is called *interstitial fluid*. Excess interstitial fluid drains into lymphatic capillaries, and is then called *lymph*. The lymph moves from lymphatic capillaries to lymphatic vessels. Ultimately, the lymphatic vessels become lymphatic ducts, which carry the lymph into veins in the lower neck (subclavian veins). Valves allow the lymph to flow in only one direction.

Lymph Nodes   Lymph nodes are located at many locations throughout the body, especially in the neck, groin, and axillary (armpit) regions. The lymph flows through the lymph nodes, which filter out pathogenic organisms and foreign chemicals.

FUNCTIONS

Return of Excess Fluid   The fluid filtered out of the capillaries each day exceeds that reabsorbed by about 3 liters. This excess is returned to the blood via the lymphatics. If this flow is blocked, there is a backup of fluid in the interstitial spaces and edema results.

Return of Protein   Most capillaries in the body have a slight permeability to protein, so there is a small, steady movement of protein from the blood into the interstitial fluid. This protein is returned to the circulatory system by the lymphatics.

Lymphatic Malfunction   When this mechanism malfunctions, fluid collects in the interstitial spaces, causing the condition known as edema (swelling). If the interstitial protein concentration increases, it alters the osmotic pressure gradient between interstitial fluid and the blood plasma, which reduces the osmotic flow at the venule end of the capillary. Decreased reabsorption of fluid into the capillary results in a build up of excess fluid—edema.

Absorption of Fat in the GI Tract   The lymphatics also provide the pathway by which fat is absorbed from the gastrointestinal tract. Lymphatic capillaries (lacteals) located in the lining of the small intestine absorb fats and fat-soluble vitamins.

Defense Mechanisms   As mentioned above, the lymph nodes filter the lymph. The nodes contain large numbers of lymphocytes and macrophages that destroy or inactivate microorganisms, foreign substances, damaged cells, and cellular debris.

LYMPH FLOW

Lymphatic vessels have one-way valves similar to those in veins. The movement of lymph through the lymphatic vessels depends on the milking action of the muscle and respiratory pumps.

LYMPHATIC VESSELS

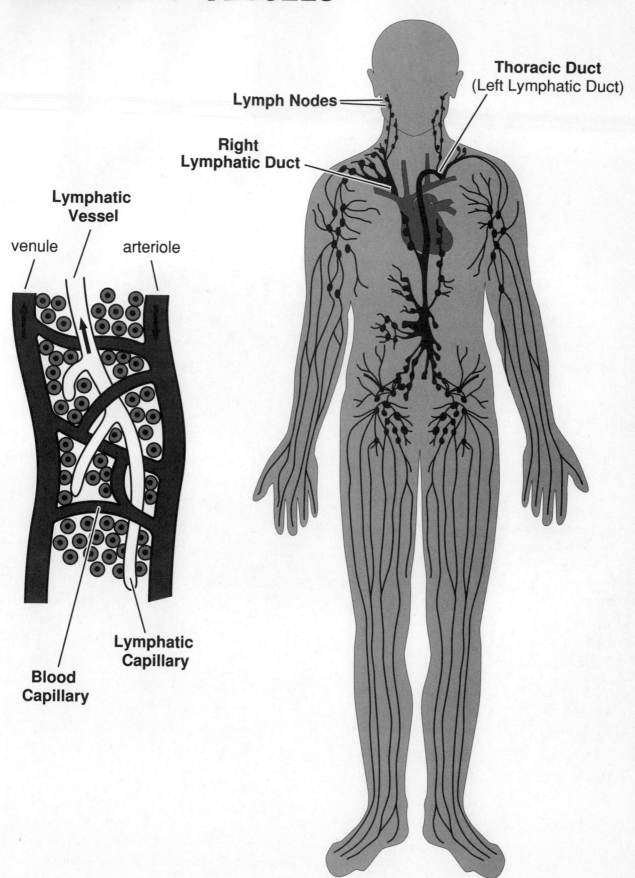

Lymph Nodes

Thoracic Duct
(Left Lymphatic Duct)

Right
Lymphatic Duct

Lymphatic
Vessel

venule   arteriole

Blood
Capillary

Lymphatic
Capillary

3 Arteries

Heart *60*
1. Right Coronary Artery
2. Left Coronary Artery

Brain *62*
1. Carotid Arteries
2. Vertebral Arteries

Upper Extremity *64*
1. Brachiocephalic Trunk
2. Subclavian
3. Axillary
4. Brachial
5. Ulnar
6. Radial
7. Superficial Palmar Arch
8. Deep Palmar Arch
9. Digitals

Aorta *66*
1. Ascending Aorta
2. Arch of Aorta
3. Thoracic Aorta
4. Abdominal Aorta

Celiac Trunk *68*
1. Common Hepatic
2. Left Gastric
3. Splenic

Superior Mesenteric Artery *70*
1. Superior Mesenteric
2. Middle Colic
3. Right Colic
4. Ileocolic
5. Jejunals
6. Ileals
7. Marginal
8. Cecal

Inferior Mesenteric Artery *72*
1. Inferior Mesenteric
2. Left Colic
3. Sigmoids
4. Superior Rectal
5. Marginal

Lower Extremity *74*
1. Common Iliac
2. Internal Iliac
3. External Iliac
4. Lateral Circumflex
5. Deep Femoral
6. Femoral
7. Descending Branch
8. Popliteal
9. Anterior Tibial
10. Posterior Tibial
11. Peroneal
12. Dorsalis Pedis
13. Plantars

ARTERIES / Heart (Coronary Arteries)

RIGHT CORONARY ARTERY

Right Coronary
> *origin :* ascending aorta (at the anterior aortic sinus of Valsalva).
> *regions supplied :* sinoatrial node, atrioventricular node, right atrium, interventricular septum, right and left ventricles.

Marginal
> *origin :* branch of the right coronary artery.
> *regions supplied :* anterior portions of the right ventricle.

Posterior Interventricular
> *origin :* posterior descending branch of the right coronary artery.
> *regions supplied :* posterior portions of the right and left ventricles.

LEFT CORONARY ARTERY

Left Coronary
> *origin :* ascending aorta (at the posterior aortic sinus of Valsalva).
> *regions supplied :* sinoatrial node, left atrium, interventricular septum, right and left ventricles.

Circumflex
> *origin :* branch of the left coronary artery.
> *regions supplied :* left atrium and posterior portions the left ventricle.

Anterior Interventricular
> *origin :* anterior descending branch of the left coronary artery.
> *regions supplied :* anterior portions of the right and left ventricles.

ARTERIES : Heart

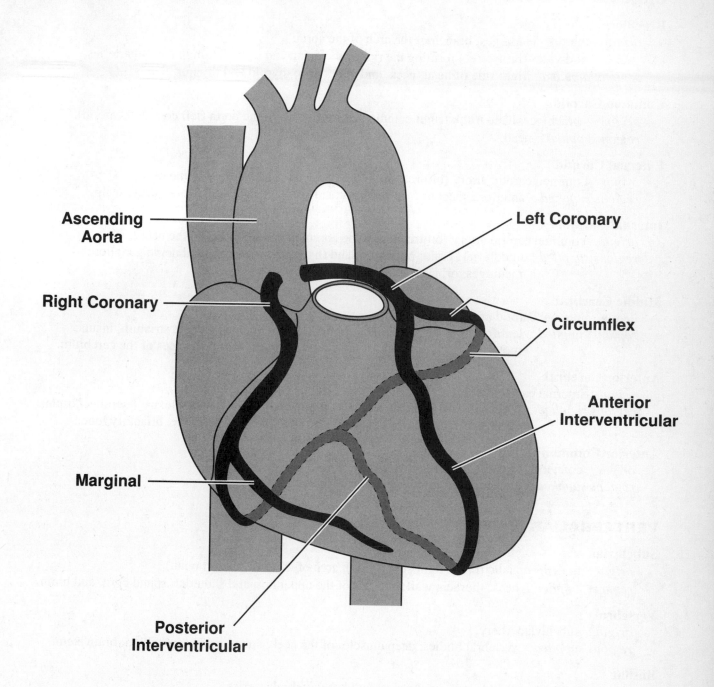

Ascending
Aorta

Right Coronary

Marginal

Left Coronary

Circumflex

Anterior
Interventricular

Posterior
Interventricular

ARTERIES / Brain

CAROTID ARTERIES

Brachiocephalic Trunk
> *origin :* the first and largest branch of the arch of the aorta;
> it divides (bifurcates) forming the right subclavian and right common carotid arteries.
> *regions supplied :* right side of head, neck, and upper arm; thyroid and thymus glands.

Common Carotid
> *origin :* brachiocephalic trunk (right common carotid); arch of the aorta (left common carotid).
> *region supplied :* head.

External Carotid
> *origin :* common carotid artery (bifurcation of the common carotid artery in the neck).
> *regions supplied :* anterior aspect of face and neck; side of the head; skull; dura mater; scalp.

Internal Carotid
> *origin :* common carotid artery (bifurcation of the common carotid artery in the neck).
> *regions supplied :* middle ear; brain; pituitary gland (hypophysis); trigeminal nerve ganglion;
> meninges; orbit (eye socket).

Middle Cerebral
> *origin :* internal carotid artery.
> *regions supplied :* lentiform nucleus; internal capsule; caudate nucleus; corpus striatum; insula;
> motor, premotor, sensory, and auditory cortex; lateral surfaces of the cerebrum.

Anterior Cerebral
> *origin :* internal carotid artery.
> *regions supplied :* hypothalamus; caudate nucleus; internal capsule; choroid plexus; lateral ventricle;
> corpus striatum; corpus callosum; frontal lobe; parietal lobe; olfactory lobe.

Anterior Communicating
> *origin :* connects the two anterior cerebral arteries.
> *regions supplied :* anterior perforated substance of the brain.

VERTEBRAL ARTERIES

Subclavian
> *origin :* brachiocephalic trunk (right subclavian); arch of aorta (left subclavian).
> *regions supplied :* neck, thoracic wall, muscles of the upper arm and shoulder, spinal cord, and brain.

Vertebral
> *origin :* subclavian artery.
> *regions supplied :* vertebral bodies; deep muscles of the neck; spinal cord; cerebellum; brain stem.

Basilar
> *origin :* formed by the junction of the right and left vertebral arteries.
> *regions supplied :* pons; internal ear; cerebellum; pineal body; ventricles; posterior part of the cerebrum.

Posterior Cerebral
> *origin :* basilar artery (terminal bifurcation).
> *regions supplied :* thalamus; globus pallidus; cerebral peduncle; colliculi; pineal body; medial and lateral
> geniculate bodies; medial and lateral occipitotemporal gyri; occipital lobe.

Posterior Communicating
> *origin :* connects the internal carotid artery with the posterior cerebral artery.
> *regions supplied :* base of the brain between the infundibulum and optic tract; internal capsule; thalamus.

ARTERIES : Brain

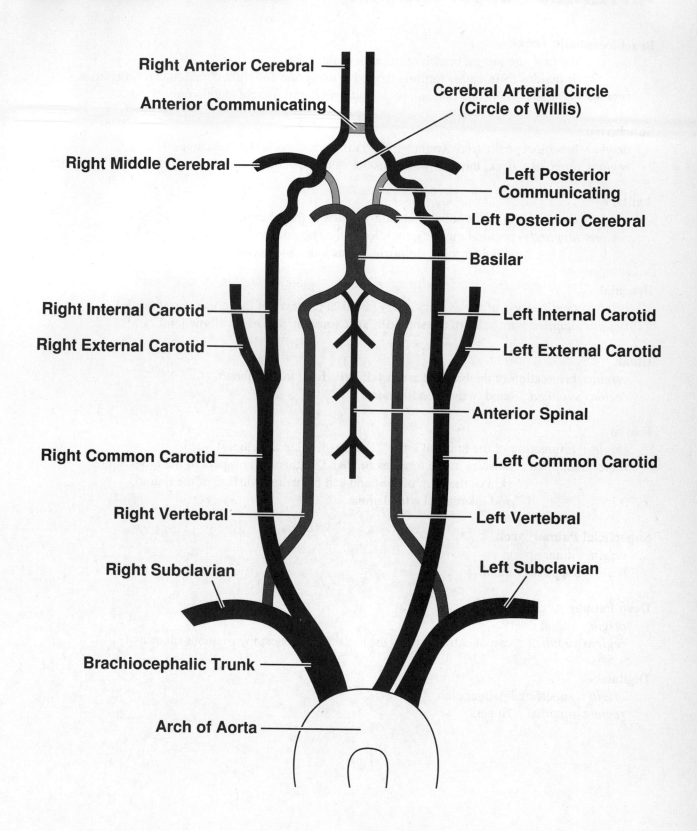

Right Anterior Cerebral

Anterior Communicating

Cerebral Arterial Circle
(Circle of Willis)

Right Middle Cerebral

Left Posterior
Communicating

Left Posterior Cerebral

Basilar

Right Internal Carotid

Left Internal Carotid

Right External Carotid

Left External Carotid

Anterior Spinal

Right Common Carotid

Left Common Carotid

Right Vertebral

Left Vertebral

Right Subclavian

Left Subclavian

Brachiocephalic Trunk

Arch of Aorta

Brachiocephalic Trunk
    origin : the first and largest branch of the arch of the aorta;
                 it divides (bifurcates) forming the right subclavian and right common carotid arteries.
    regions supplied : right side of head, neck, and upper arm; thyroid and thymus glands.

Subclavian
    origin : brachiocephalic trunk (right subclavian); arch of aorta (left subclavian).
    regions supplied : neck, thoracic wall, muscles of the upper arm and shoulder, spinal cord, and brain.

Axillary
    origin : continuation of the subclavian artery (starts at the outer border of the 1st rib).
    regions supplied : pectoral muscles, muscles of the shoulder and upper arm, acromion,
                 shoulder joint, sternoclavicular joint, and breast.

Brachial
    origin : continuation of the axillary artery (starts at the level of the teres major muscle)
    regions supplied : muscles of the shoulder, arm, forearm, and hand; elbow joint.

Ulnar
    origin : bifurcation of the brachial artery (slightly distal to the elbow).
    regions supplied : hand, wrist, and forearm.

Radial
    origin : bifurcation of the brachial artery (slightly distal to the elbow).
    regions supplied : muscles of the forearm and hand, radius, outer aspect of the index finger,
                 skin of the back of the hand and the palmar surface of the thumb,
                 and intercarpal articulations.

Superficial Palmar Arch
    origin : ulnar artery.
    regions supplied : palm.

Deep Palmar Arch
    origin : radial artery.
    regions supplied : carpal extremities of the metacarpal bones; interosseous muscles.

Digitals
    origin : superficial palmar arch.
    regions supplied : fingers.

ARTERIES : Right Upper Extremity

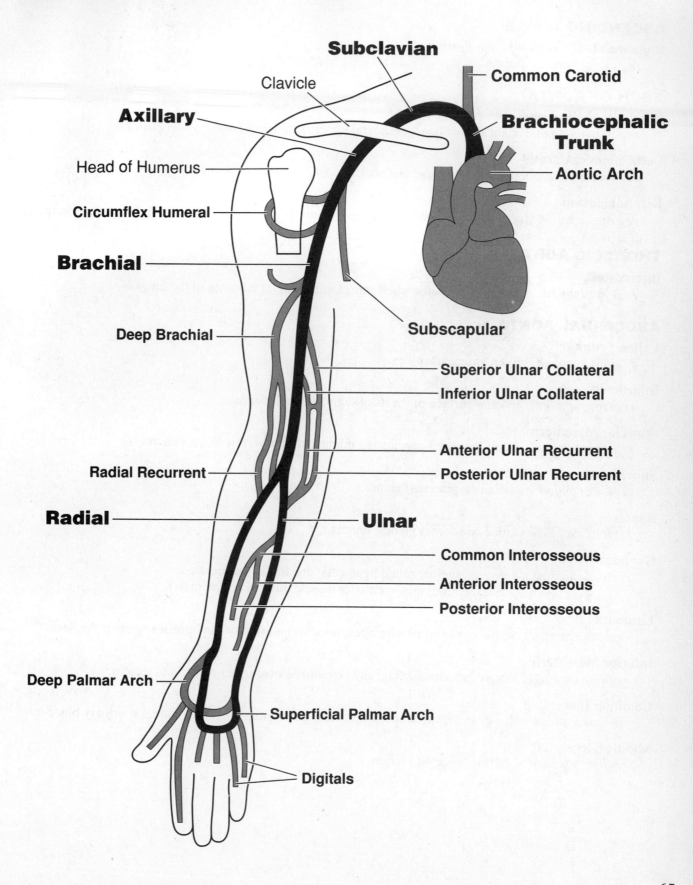

Subclavian

Clavicle

Common Carotid

Axillary

Brachiocephalic Trunk

Head of Humerus

Aortic Arch

Circumflex Humeral

Brachial

Deep Brachial

Subscapular

Superior Ulnar Collateral

Inferior Ulnar Collateral

Anterior Ulnar Recurrent

Radial Recurrent

Posterior Ulnar Recurrent

Radial

Ulnar

Common Interosseous

Anterior Interosseous

Posterior Interosseous

Deep Palmar Arch

Superficial Palmar Arch

Digitals

ARTERIES / Aorta

ASCENDING AORTA

Right and Left Coronary (not illustrated)
region supplied :   heart.

ARCH OF AORTA

Brachiocephalic Trunk
regions supplied :   right side of head, neck, and upper arm; thyroid and thymus glands.

Left Common Carotid
region supplied : left side of the head and neck.

Left Subclavian
regions supplied : neck, thoracic wall, muscles of the upper arm and shoulder, spinal cord, and brain.

THORACIC AORTA

Intercostals
region supplied : intercostal muscles; chest muscles; pleural membranes of the lungs.

ABDOMINAL AORTA

Celiac Trunk
regions supplied : liver, stomach, spleen.

Inferior Phrenics
regions supplied : inferior surface of the diaphragm; adrenal glands.

Superior Mesenteric
regions supplied : small intestine; cecum; ascending and transverse colons; pancreas.

Suprarenals
region supplied : adrenal (suprarenal) glands.

Renals
regions supplied : kidneys; adrenal glands; ureters.

Gonadals
regions supplied :   ovaries; uterus; round ligaments; ureters (in the female).
testes; epididymis; cremaster muscle; ureters (in the male).

Lumbars
regions supplied : spinal cord and its meninges; muscles and skin of the lumbar region of the back.

Inferior Mesenteric
regions supplied : transverse, descending, and sigmoid colons; upper part of the rectum.

Common Iliacs
regions supplied : lower extremities; uterus; prostate gland; muscles of the buttocks; urinary bladder.

Middle Sacral
regions supplied : sacrum; coccyx; rectum.

ARTERIES : Aorta and Its Major Branches

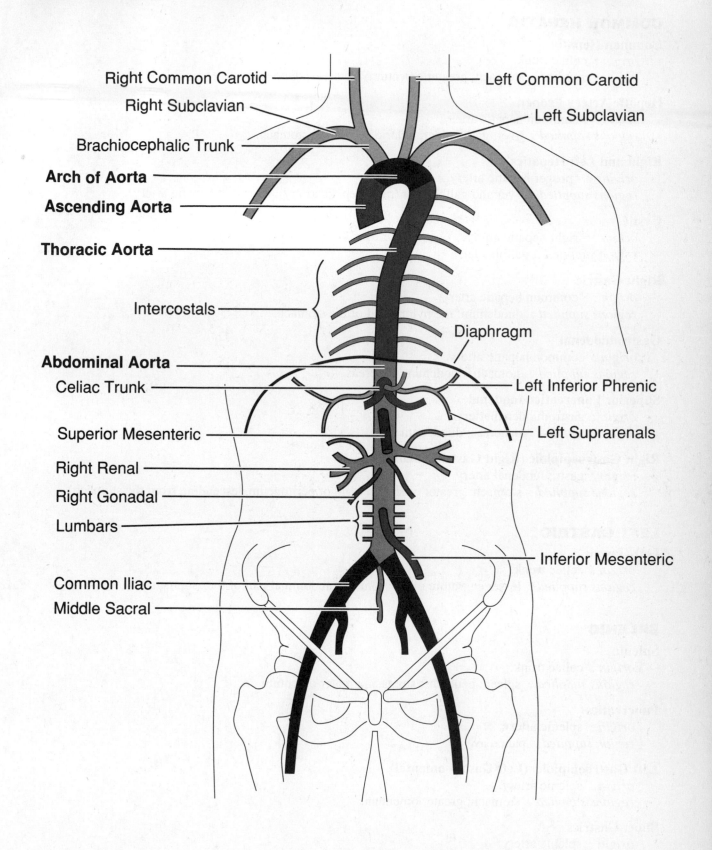

Right Common Carotid

Right Subclavian

Brachiocephalic Trunk

Arch of Aorta

Ascending Aorta

Thoracic Aorta

Intercostals

Abdominal Aorta

Celiac Trunk

Superior Mesenteric

Right Renal

Right Gonadal

Lumbars

Common Iliac

Middle Sacral

Left Common Carotid

Left Subclavian

Diaphragm

Left Inferior Phrenic

Left Suprarenals

Inferior Mesenteric

ARTERIES / Celiac Trunk

COMMON HEPATIC

Common Hepatic
origin : celiac trunk
regions supplied : stomach; greater omentum; pancreas; duodenum; liver; gallbladder.

Hepatic Artery Proper
origin : common hepatic artery.
regions supplied : liver; gallbladder; pyloric part of the stomach.

Right and Left Hepatics
origins : proper hepatic artery.
regions supplied : liver and gallbladder (right hepatic artery); liver (left hepatic artery).

Cystic
origin : right hepatic artery.
region supplied : gallbladder.

Right Gastric
origin : common hepatic artery.
regions supplied : duodenum; the pyloric end of the stomach.

Gastroduodenal
origin : common hepatic artery.
regions supplied : stomach; duodenum; pancreas.

Superior Pancreaticoduodenal
origin : gastroduodenal artery.
regions supplied : pancreas; duodenum.

Right Gastroepiploic (Right Gastro-omental)
origin : gastroduodenal artery.
regions supplied : stomach; greater omentum (fold of peritoneum descending from the stomach).

LEFT GASTRIC

Left Gastric
origin : celiac trunk.
regions supplied : lesser curvature of the stomach; abdominal part of the esophagus.

SPLENIC

Splenic
origin : celiac trunk.
regions supplied : spleen; pancreas; stomach; greater omentum.

Pancreatics
origin : splenic artery.
region supplied : pancreas.

Left Gastroepiploic (Left Gastro-omental)
origin : splenic artery.
regions supplied : stomach; greater omentum.

Short Gastrics
origin : splenic artery.
regions supplied : fundus (upper portion) of the stomach.

ARTERIES : Celiac Trunk

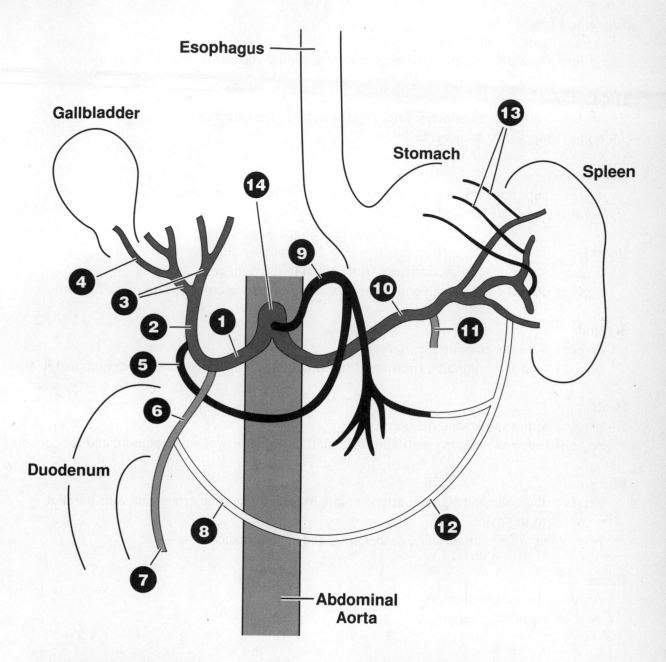

Esophagus

Gallbladder

Stomach

Spleen

Duodenum

Abdominal
Aorta

(1) Common Hepatic
(2) Hepatic Artery Proper
(3) Right & Left Hepatics
(4) Cystic
(5) Right gastric
(6) Gastroduodenal
(7) Superior Pancreaticoduodenal
(8) Right Gastroepiploic

(9) Left Gastric
(10) Splenic
(11) Great Pancreatic
(12) Left Gastroepiploic
(13) Short Gastrics
(14) Celiac Trunk

Superior Mesenteric
origin : abdominal aorta.
regions supplied : small intestine; cecum; ascending and transverse colons; pancreas.

Middle Colic
origin : superior mesenteric artery (just caudal to the pancreas).
regions supplied : transverse colon.

Right Colic
origin : superior mesenteric artery (just caudal to the middle colic artery).
regions supplied : ascending colon.

Ileocolic
origin : superior mesenteric artery (just caudal to the right colic artery).
regions supplied : cecum; vermiform appendix; ascending colon; distal part of ileum.

Jejunals
origin : superior mesenteric artery.
regions supplied : jejunum (portion of the small intestine between the duodenum and ileum).

Ileals
origin : superior mesenteric artery.
regions supplied : ileum (portion of the small intestine between the jejunum and the cecum).

Marginal
origin : the colic and sigmoid arteries unite to form a marginal artery that runs parallel to the colon.
regions supplied : transverse, descending, and sigmoid colons.

Cecal
origin : the marginal artery.
regions supplied : cecum.

ARTERIES : Superior Mesenteric

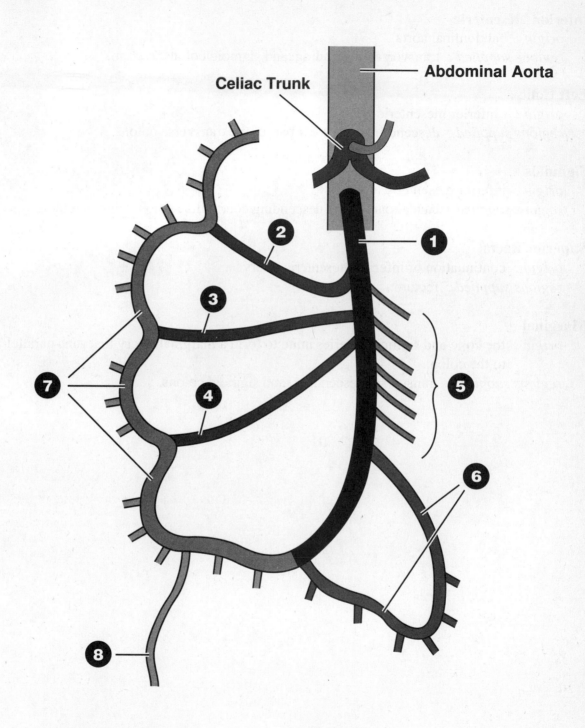

Abdominal Aorta

Celiac Trunk

(1) Superior Mesenteric
(2) Middle Colic
(3) Right Colic
(4) Ileocolic
(5) Jejunals
(6) Ileals
(7) Marginal
(8) Cecal

Inferior Mesenteric
origin : abdominal aorta
regions supplied : transverse, descending, and sigmoid colons; rectum.

Left Colic
origin : inferior mesenteric artery.
regions supplied : descending colon; left part of the transverse colon.

Sigmoids
origin : inferior mesenteric artery.
regions supplied : caudal part of the descending colon; iliac colon; sigmoid colon.

Superior Rectal
origin : continuation of inferior mesenteric artery.
regions supplied : rectum.

Marginal
origin : the colic and sigmoid arteries unite to form a marginal artery that runs parallel to the colon.
regions supplied : transverse, descending, and sigmoid colons.

ARTERIES : Inferior Mesenteric

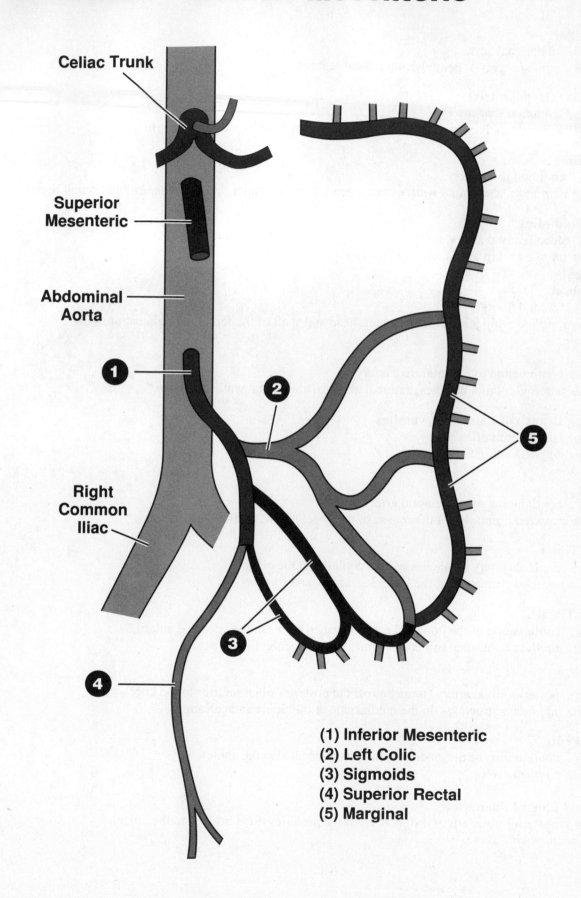

Celiac Trunk

Superior Mesenteric

Abdominal Aorta

Right Common Iliac

(1) Inferior Mesenteric
(2) Left Colic
(3) Sigmoids
(4) Superior Rectal
(5) Marginal

ARTERIES / Lower Extremity

Common Iliac
origin :   abdominal aorta.
regions supplied : pelvis, genitals, and gluteal regions.

Internal Iliac (Hypogastric)
origin :   common iliac artery.
regions supplied : pelvis, external genitals, anus, and medial aspect of the thigh.

External Iliac
origin : common iliac artery.
regions supplied : abdominal wall, external genitals, psoas major, ductus deferens, and round ligament.

Lateral Circumflex
origin : deep femoral artery.
regions supplied : hip joint and thigh muscles.

Deep Femoral
origin : femoral artery.
regions supplied : hip joint, thigh muscles, head and shaft of the femur, and gluteal muscles.

Femoral
origin : continuation of external iliac artery.
regions supplied : thigh muscles, external genitals, abdominal wall, and groin.

Descending Branch of Lateral Circumflex
origin : lateral circumflex artery.
regions supplied : thigh.

Popliteal
origin : continuation of the femoral artery.
regions supplied : muscles in the region of the knee, femur, patella, and tibia.

Anterior Tibial
origin : popliteal artery (branches off the popliteal in the calf).
regions supplied : muscles of the knee, leg, ankle, and foot.

Posterior Tibial
origin : continuation of the popliteal artery (located between the knee and ankle).
regions supplied : muscles and bones of the leg, ankle, and foot.

Peroneal
origin : posterior tibial artery (branches off the posterior tibial inferior to the knee).
regions supplied : structures on the medial side of the fibula and calcaneus.

Dorsalis Pedis
origin : continuation of the anterior tibial artery (located at the ankle).
regions supplied : foot.

Medial and Lateral Plantars
origin : posterior tibial artery (bifurcation of the posterior tibial inferior to the ankle).
regions supplied : foot.

ARTERIES : Lower Extremity

Anterior View

Posterior View

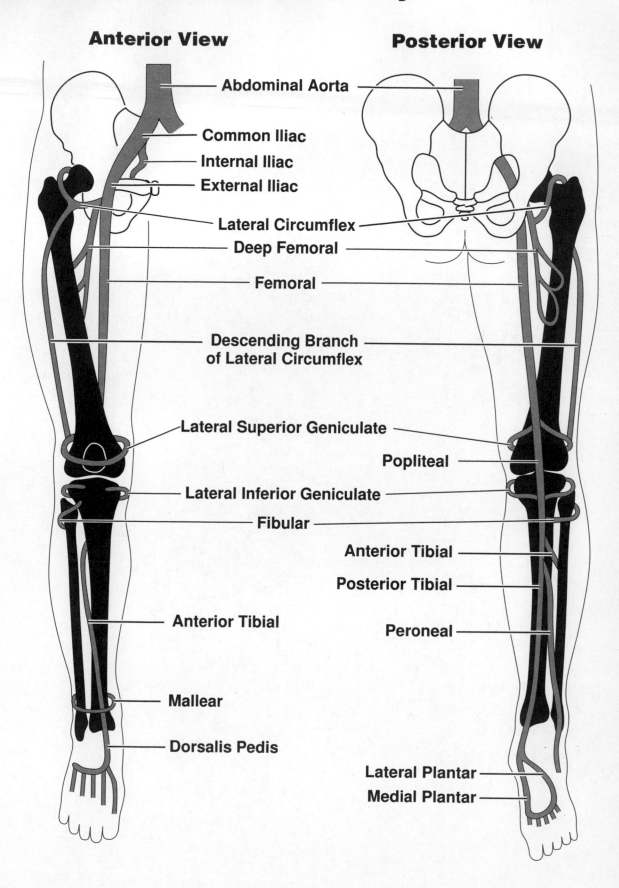

- Abdominal Aorta
- Common Iliac
- Internal Iliac
- External Iliac
- Lateral Circumflex
- Deep Femoral
- Femoral
- Descending Branch of Lateral Circumflex
- Lateral Superior Geniculate
- Popliteal
- Lateral Inferior Geniculate
- Fibular
- Anterior Tibial
- Posterior Tibial
- Anterior Tibial
- Peroneal
- Mallear
- Dorsalis Pedis
- Lateral Plantar
- Medial Plantar

4 Veins

Heart (Coronary Veins) 78
1. Small Cardiac Vein
2. Smallest Cardiac Veins
3. Anterior Cardiac Veins
4. Middle Cardiac Vein
5. Great Cardiac Vein
6. Coronary Sinus

Brain and Face 80
1. Superior Sagittal Sinus
2. Occipital Sinus
3. Inferior Sagittal Sinus
4. Straight Sinus
5. Transverse Sinuses
6. Sigmoid Sinuses
7. Internal Jugular Veins
8. External Jugular Veins

Upper Extremity 82
Superficial Veins
1. Median Antebrachial   2. Cephalic   3. Basilic   4. Median Cubital

Deep Veins
5. Radial
6. Ulnar
7. Brachial
8. Axillary
9. Subclavian
10. Brachiocephalic
11. Superior Vena Cava

Inferior Vena Cava 84
1. Internal Iliacs
2. External Iliacs
3. Common Iliacs
4. Lumbars
5. Gonadals
6. Renals
7. Suprarenals
8. Hepatics
9. Inferior Phrenics

Azygos System 86
1. Common Iliacs
2. Ascending Lumbars
3. Lumbars
4. Right Highest Intercostal
5. Left Superior Intercostal
6. Posterior Intercostal
7. Hemiazygos
8. Accessory Hemiazygos
9. Esophageals
10. Mediastinals
11. Pericardials
12. Bronchials
13. Azygos

Hepatic Portal System 88
1. Superior Mesenteric   2. Splenic   3. Hepatic Portal

Lower Extremity 90
Superficial Veins
1. Dorsal Venous Arch   2. Great Saphenous   3. Small Saphenous

Deep Veins
4. Plantar Venous Arch
5. Plantars
6. Peroneal
7. Posterior Tibial
8. Dorsalis Pedis
9. Anterior Tibial
10. Popliteal
11. Femoral
12. Internal Iliac
13. External Iliac
14. Common Iliac

VEINS / Heart (Coronary Veins)

Small Cardiac Vein
location :   ascends up the back of the heart from the back of the right atrium and ventricle.
drains :   back of the right atrium and ventricle; right marginal vein.
empties into : right extremity of the coronary sinus or the right atrium.

Smallest Cardiac Veins   (many minute veins)
location :   in the muscular wall of the heart.
drains :   muscular wall of the heart.
empties into : mostly into atria; some into ventricles.

Anterior Cardiac Veins   (3 or 4 in number)
location :   ventral side of the heart.
drains :   ventral side of the right ventricle.
empties into : right atrium.

Middle Cardiac Vein
location :   ascends up the back of the heart from the apex.
drains : tributaries from both ventricles.
empties into : right extremity of the coronary sinus.

Great Cardiac Vein
location :   from the apex of the heart it ascends to the front of the heart.
drains : tributaries from the left atrium and both ventricles; left marginal vein.
empties into : left extremity of the coronary sinus.

Coronary Sinus   (wide venous channel about 2.25 cm in length)
location :   posterior part of the coronary sulcus (covered by muscular fibers from the atrium).
drains : great, small, and middle cardiac veins; posterior vein of left ventricle; oblique vein of left atrium.
empties into : right atrium (between the opening of the inferior vena cava and the atrioventricular
                   aperture).

VEINS : Heart

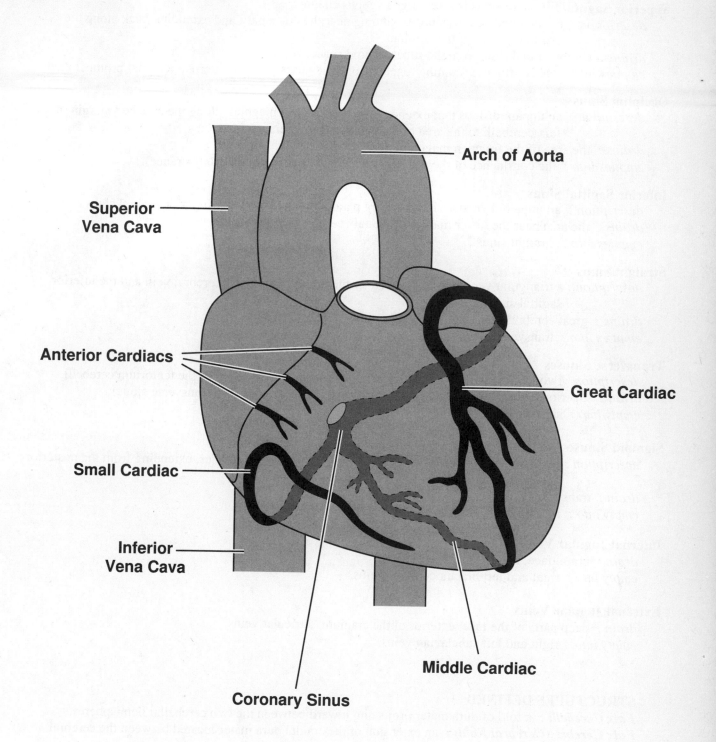

Arch of Aorta

Superior Vena Cava

Anterior Cardiacs

Great Cardiac

Small Cardiac

Inferior Vena Cava

Middle Cardiac

Coronary Sinus

VEINS / Brain and Face

Superior Sagittal Sinus (a sinus is an enlarged venous channel)
   description : an unpaired venous sinus beginning near the crista galli and extending back along the sagittal groove of the cranium.
   drains : cerebrospinal fluid from the subarachnoid space.
   empties into : the confluence (coming together) of the sinuses near the internal occipital protuberance.

Occipital Sinus
   description : an unpaired sinus that extends from the foramen magnum along the attached margin of the falx cerebelli to the area of the occipital protuberance.
   drains : the area of the foramen magnum.
   empties into : the confluence of the sinuses (near the internal occipital protuberance).

Inferior Sagittal Sinus
   description : an unpaired venous sinus running parallel to and below the superior sagittal sinus.
   drains : the area near the lower margin of the falx cerebri (cerebral fold).
   empties into : straight sinus.

Straight Sinus
   description : a triangular venous sinus formed by the union of the great cerebral vein and the inferior sagittal sinus.
   drains : great cerebral vein; inferior sagittal sinus; cerebellar veins.
   empties into : transverse sinus.

Transverse Sinuses
   description : two large venous sinuses located along the attached margin of the tentorium cerebelli.
   drain : superior sagittal sinus (right transverse sinus); straight sinus (left transverse sinus).
   empty into : sigmoid sinuses.

Sigmoid Sinuses
   description : S-shaped continuations of the right and left transverse sinuses, extending from the posterior surface of the temporal bone to the jugular foramen.
   drain : transverse sinuses.
   empty into : right and left internal jugular veins.

Internal Jugular Veins
   drain : brain, face, and neck.
   empty into : right and left brachiocephalic veins.

External Jugular Veins
   drain : deep parts of the face; exterior of the cranium; auricular veins.
   empty into : right and left subclavian veins.

STRUCTURES DEFINED
Falx Cerebelli : a fold of dura mater projecting inward between the two cerebellar hemispheres.
Falx Cerebri (Cerebral Fold) : an extension of the cranial dura mater located between the cerebral hemispheres; it encloses the superior and inferior sagittal sinuses.
Tentorium Cerebelli : a transverse shelf of dura mater that forms a partition between the occipital lobes of the cerebral hemispheres and the cerebellum.

VEINS : Brain and Face

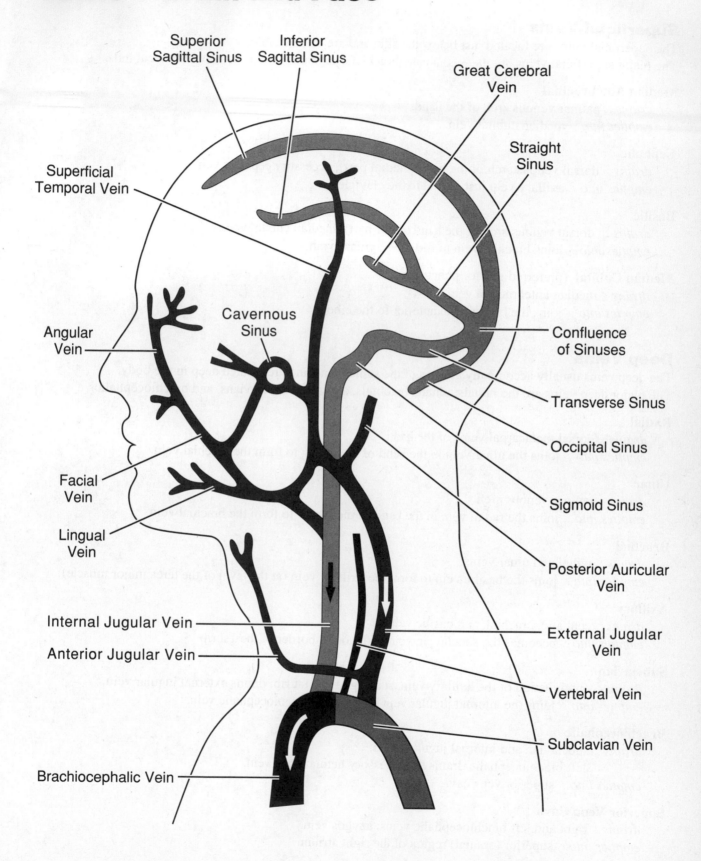

Superior Sagittal Sinus

Inferior Sagittal Sinus

Great Cerebral Vein

Straight Sinus

Superficial Temporal Vein

Cavernous Sinus

Confluence of Sinuses

Angular Vein

Transverse Sinus

Occipital Sinus

Facial Vein

Sigmoid Sinus

Lingual Vein

Posterior Auricular Vein

Internal Jugular Vein

External Jugular Vein

Anterior Jugular Vein

Vertebral Vein

Subclavian Vein

Brachiocephalic Vein

VEINS / Upper Extremity

Superficial Veins

The superficial veins are located just below the skin and are often visible.
The major superficial veins are the median antebrachials, cephalics, basilics, and median cubitals.

Median Antebrachial
> *drains :* palmar venous arch of the hand.
> *empties into :* median cubital vein.

Cephalic
> *drains :* dorsal venous arch of the hand (medial part); accessory cephalic vein.
> *empties into :* axillary vein just caudal to the clavicle.

Basilic
> *drains :* dorsal venous arch of the hand (ulnar part); median cubital vein.
> *empties into :* joins brachial vein to form the axillary vein.

Median Cubital (preferred site for punctures)
> *drains :* median antebrachial vein.
> *empties into :* joins the basilic vein anterior to the elbow.

Deep Veins

The deep veins usually accompany arteries of the same name and are located deep in the body.
The major deep veins are the radials, ulnars, brachials, axillaries, subclavians, and brachiocephalics.

Radial
> *drains :* dorsal metacarpal veins of the hand.
> *empties into :* joins the ulnar vein in the bend of the elbow to form the brachial vein.

Ulnar
> *drains :* palmar venous arch.
> *empties into :* joins the radial vein in the bend of the elbow to form the brachial vein.

Brachial
> *drains :* radial and ulnar veins.
> *empties into :* joins the basilic vein to form the axillary vein (at the level of the teres major muscle).

Axillary
> *drains :* cephalic, brachial, and basilic veins.
> *empties into :* becomes the subclavian vein at the outer border of the 1st rib.

Subclavian
> *drains :* continuation of the axillary vein, starting at the 1st rib; drains external jugular vein.
> *empties into :* joins the internal jugular vein to form the brachiocephalic vein.

Brachiocephalic
> *drains :* subclavian and internal jugular veins;
> left brachiocephalic drains the accessory hemiazygos vein.
> *empties into :* superior vena cava.

Superior Vena Cava
> *drains :* right and left brachiocephalic veins; azygos vein.
> *empties into :* superior (cranial) region of the right atrium.

VEINS : Upper Extremity

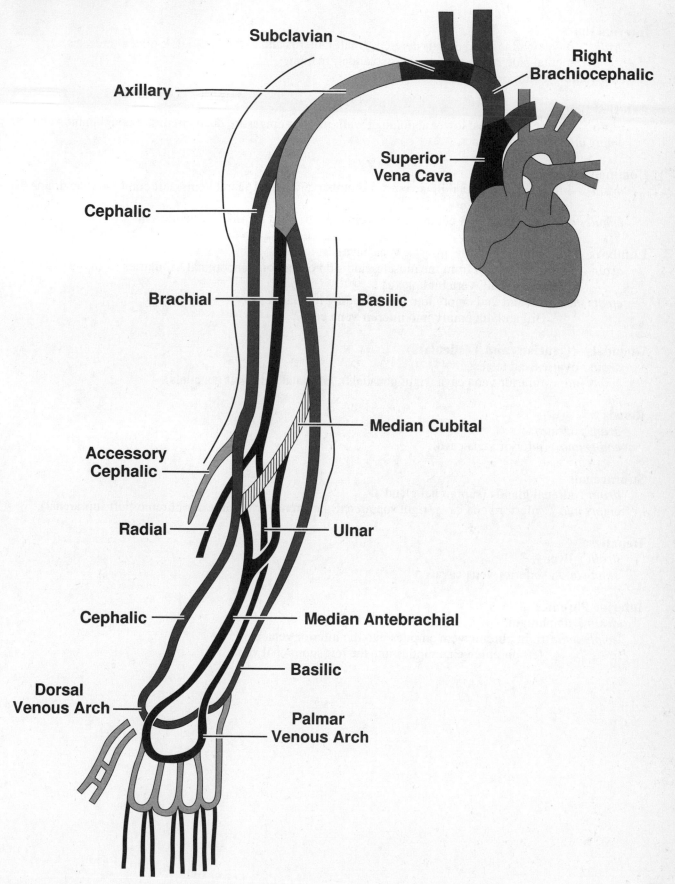

Subclavian

Axillary

Right Brachiocephalic

Superior Vena Cava

Cephalic

Brachial

Basilic

Median Cubital

Accessory Cephalic

Radial

Ulnar

Cephalic

Median Antebrachial

Basilic

Dorsal Venous Arch

Palmar Venous Arch

Internal Iliacs
drain : prostate gland and ductus deferens (male); uterus and vagina (female); gluteal muscles; medial side of the thigh; urinary bladder; rectum.
empty into : common iliacs.

External Iliacs
drain : lower extremities; lower abdominal wall; inferior epigastric deep circumflex, and pubic veins.
empty into : common iliacs.

Common Iliacs
drains : internal and external iliac veins; iliolumbar and lateral sacral veins; left common iliac drains the middle sacral vein.
empties into : left and right common iliac veins join to form the inferior vena cava.

Lumbars (4 on each side of the inferior vena cava)
drain : dorsal tributaries from the muscles and skin of the loin; abdominal tributaries from the abdominal wall; vertebral plexus.
empty into : 1st and 2nd empty into the ascending lumbar vein;
3rd and 4th empty into inferior vena cava.

Gonadals (Ovarians and Testiculars)
drain : ovaries and testes.
empty into : inferior vena cava (right gonadals); left renal vein (left gonadals).

Renals
drain : kidneys.
empty into : inferior vena cava.

Suprarenals
drain : adrenal glands (suprarenal glands).
empty into : inferior vena cava (right suprarenal); left renal or left inferior phrenic (left suprarenal).

Hepatics
drain : liver.
empty into : inferior vena cava.

Inferior Phrenics
drain : diaphragm.
empty into: right phrenic vein empties into the inferior vena cava;
left phrenic vein empties into the left suprarenal vein.

VEINS : Inferior Vena Cava and Its Tributaries

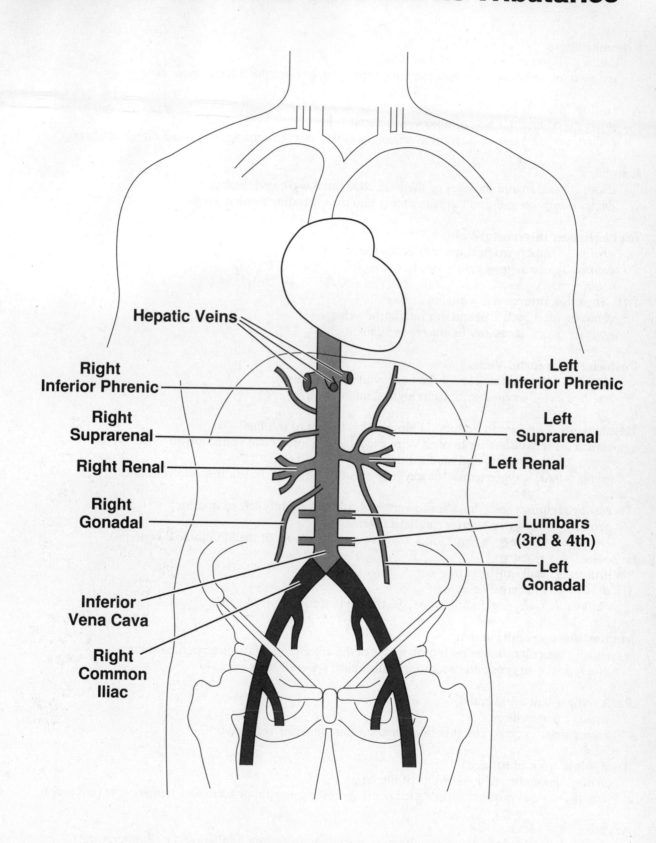

Hepatic Veins

Right
Inferior Phrenic

Left
Inferior Phrenic

Right
Suprarenal

Left
Suprarenal

Right Renal

Left Renal

Right
Gonadal

Lumbars
(3rd & 4th)

Left
Gonadal

Inferior
Vena Cava

Right
Common
Iliac

Common Iliacs
drain : internal and external iliac veins.
empty into : right and left common iliac veins join to form the inferior vena cava.

Ascending Lumbars
drain : common iliacs; lumbar veins; sacral veins.
empty into : azygos vein (right ascending lumbar); hemiazygos vein (left ascending lumbar).

Lumbars
drain : the skin and muscles of the loin; abdominal wall; vertebral plexus.
empty into : 1st and 2nd lumbars empty into the ascending lumbar veins.

Right Highest Intercostal Vein
drains : upper two or three intercostal spaces.
empties into : azygos vein.

Left Superior Intercostal Vein
drains : left 2nd, 3rd, and 4th intercostal veins.
empties into : accessory hemiazygos vein.

Posterior Intercostal Veins
drain : skin and muscles of the back; vertebral plexuses.
empties into : azygos vein; right highest intercostal.

Hemiazygos (anterior to vertebral column, slightly left of midline)
drains : left ascending lumbar vein; caudal 4 or 5 intercostal veins; left subcostal vein; esophageal and mediastinal veins.
empties into: azygos (joins the azygos vein at the level of the 9th thoracic vertebra).

Accessory Hemiazygos (anterior to vertebral column, slightly left of midline)
drains : 4th to 7th posterior intercostal veins.
empties into : azygos vein (joins azygos vein at the level of the 8th thoracic vertebra).

Esophageals (not illustrated)
drain : esophagus.
empty into : azygos, hemiazygos, gastric, and inferior thyroid veins.

Mediastinals (not illustrated)
drain : aereolar tissue and lymph nodes of the anterior mediastinum; pericardium.
empty into : azygos and brachiocephalic veins; superior vena cava

Pericardials (not illustrated)
drain : pericardium.
empty into : azygos and brachiocephalic veins; superior vena cava.

Bronchials (not illustrated)
drain : larger bronchi and roots of the lungs.
empty into : azygos vein (right side); left highest intercostal or accessory hemiazygos (left side).

Azygos
drains : hemiazygos; accessory hemiazygos; right ascending lumbar; and right intercostals.
empties into : superior vena cava.

VEINS : Azygos System

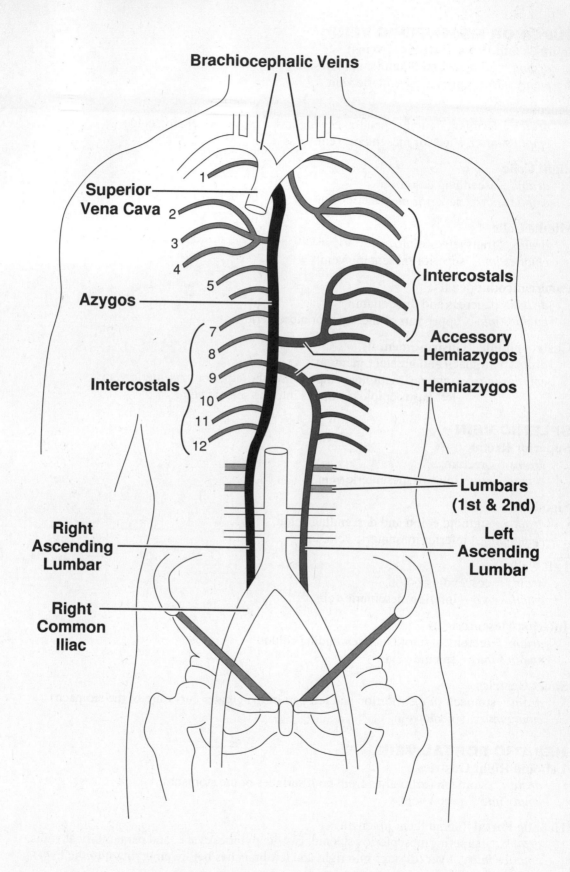

Brachiocephalic Veins

Superior Vena Cava

1

2

3

4

5

Azygos

7

8

9

Intercostals

10

11

12

Intercostals

Accessory Hemiazygos

Hemiazygos

Lumbars (1st & 2nd)

Right Ascending Lumbar

Left Ascending Lumbar

Right Common Iliac

VEINS / Hepatic Portal System

SUPERIOR MESENTERIC VEIN

Jejunals and Ileals (intestinal veins)
drain : jejunum and ileum (small intestine).
empty into : superior mesenteric vein.

Ileocolic
drains : terminal ileum; appendix; cecum; lower part of ascending colon.
empties into : superior mesenteric vein.

Right Colic
drains : ascending colon.
empties into : superior mesenteric vein.

Middle Colic
drains : transverse colon.
empties into: superior mesenteric vein.

Pancreaticoduodenal
drains: pancreas and duodenum.
empties into : upper part of the superior mesenteric vein.

Gastroepiploic (Gastro-omental)
drains : stomach and greater omentum.
empties into : right gastroepiploic empties into the superior mesenteric vein;
left gastroepiploic empties into the splenic vein.

SPLENIC VEIN

Superior Rectal
drains : rectum.
empties into : inferior mesenteric vein.

Sigmoids
drain : sigmoid colon and descending colon.
empty into : inferior mesenteric vein.

Left Colic
drains : descending colon.
empties into : inferior mesenteric vein.

Inferior Mesenteric
drains : rectum; sigmoid and descending colons.
empties into : splenic vein.

Short Gastrics
drain : stomach (upper portion and left part of the greater curvature of the stomach).
empty into : splenic vein.

HEPATIC PORTAL VEIN

Left and Right Gastrics
drain : stomach (tributaries from both surfaces of the stomach).
empty into : portal vein.

Hepatic Portal (about 8 cm in length)
drains : superior mesenteric , splenic, gastric, pyloric, cystic, and paraumbilical veins.
empties into : liver (divides into right and left branches before emptying into the liver).

VEINS : Hepatic Portal System

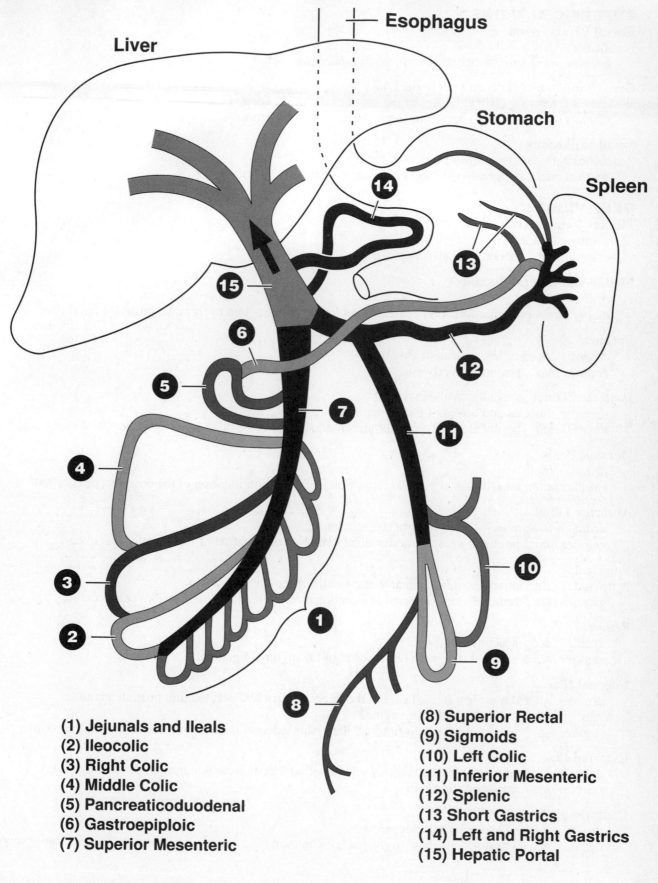

Liver

Esophagus

Stomach

Spleen

(1) Jejunals and Ileals
(2) Ileocolic
(3) Right Colic
(4) Middle Colic
(5) Pancreaticoduodenal
(6) Gastroepiploic
(7) Superior Mesenteric

(8) Superior Rectal
(9) Sigmoids
(10) Left Colic
(11) Inferior Mesenteric
(12) Splenic
(13 Short Gastrics
(14) Left and Right Gastrics
(15) Hepatic Portal

VEINS / Lower Extremity

SUPERFICIAL VEINS
Dorsal Venous Arch
drains : foot
empties into : great saphenous vein; small saphenous vein.

Great Saphenous   (longest vein in the body)
drains : foot; superficial tissues of the lower extremities; deep veins.
empties into : femoral vein (joins the femoral vein in the groin).

Small Saphenous
drains : foot and posterior portion of the leg.
empties into : popliteal vein (joins popliteal vein behind the knee).

DEEP VEINS
Plantar Venous Arch
drains : foot.
empties into : medial and lateral plantar veins.

Medial and Lateral Plantars
drain : foot.
empty into : posterior tibial vein (medial and lateral plantars join to form the posterior tibial vein).

Peroneal
drains : leg muscles; calcaneus (heel).
empties into : posterior tibial vein.

Posterior Tibial   (usually two veins)
drains : muscles and bones of the posterior leg.
empties into : popliteal vein (posterior and anterior tibial veins unite to form the popliteal vein).

Dorsalis Pedis
drains : foot.
empties into : anterior tibial vein (anterior tibial vein is a continuation of the dorsalis pedis veins).

Anterior Tibial
drains : foot; muscles and bones of the anterior leg.
empties into : popliteal vein   (anterior tibial vein is a continuation of the dorsalis pedis veins).

Popliteal
drains : anterior and posterior tibial veins; small saphenous vein.
empties into : femoral vein (femoral is a continuation of the popliteal just above the knee).

Femoral
drains : deep structures of the thigh.
empties into : external iliac vein (at the level of the inguinal ligament).

Internal Iliac
drains : gluteal muscles; medial side of the thigh; urinary bladder; rectum; prostate gland;
          ductus deferens; uterus; vagina.
empties into : common iliac vein (internal iliac joins external iliac to form the common iliac vein).

External Iliac
drains : femoral vein; great saphenous vein (external iliac is a continuation of the femoral vein).
empties into : common iliac vein

Common Iliac
drains : internal and external iliac veins.
empties into : inferior vena cava (right and left common iliac veins join to form the inferior vena cava).

VEINS : Lower Extremity

Anterior View

Posterior View

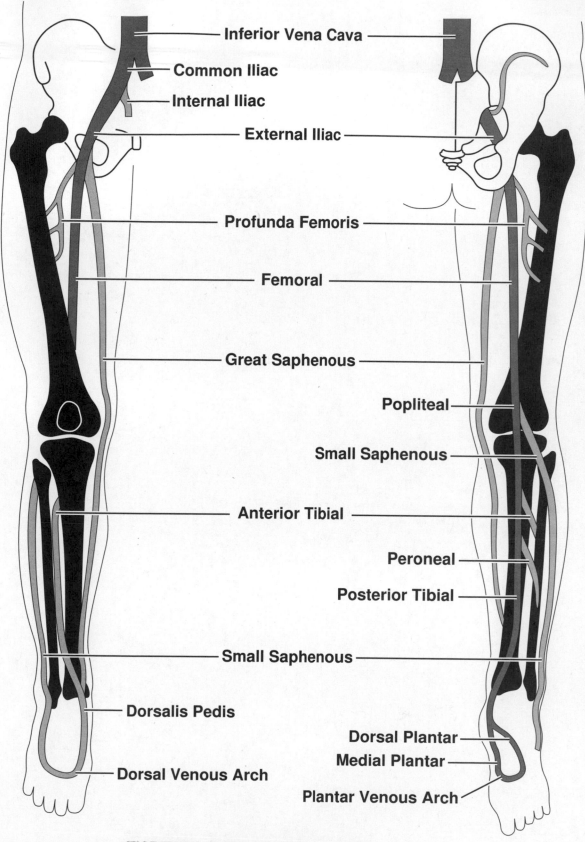

Inferior Vena Cava

Common Iliac

Internal Iliac

External Iliac

Profunda Femoris

Femoral

Great Saphenous

Popliteal

Small Saphenous

Anterior Tibial

Peroneal

Posterior Tibial

Small Saphenous

Dorsalis Pedis

Dorsal Plantar

Medial Plantar

Dorsal Venous Arch

Plantar Venous Arch

5 Blood

BLOOD / Composition : Overview

Blood is composed of two portions : plasma and formed elements. The plasma is a watery liquid containing many dissolved substances. The formed elements are cells and cell fragments.

PLASMA
Water
Plasma is approximately 91.5% water and 8.5% solutes (dissolved substances).

Plasma Proteins
About 70% of the solutes are proteins. The three main types of plasma proteins are albumins, globulins (include antibodies), and coagulation factors (such as fibrinogen).

Nonprotein Organic Compounds
About 20% of the solutes are small organic molecules. They include nutrients, metabolic wastes (nitrogen-containing compounds), and organic acids. Hormones make up a very small portion of this group of compounds.

Inorganic Components
About 10% of the solutes are inorganic salts, buffers, and gases.

FORMED ELEMENTS
Red Blood Cells (RBCs)   also called erythrocytes
Concentration   5 – 6.5 million / mm^3.
Erythrocytes make up 45% of the total blood volume in men and 42% in women. The percentage of the total blood volume occupied by red blood cells is called the hematocrit.
Size and Shape   The diameter of a red blood cell is 7 micrometers, just small enough to squeeze through a capillary. These cells have the shape of a biconcave disc.
Function   The major function of these cells is to carry oxygen and carbon dioxide between the lungs and the body tissues. The iron-containing protein hemoglobin facilitates the transport of oxygen; an enzyme called carbonic anhydrase facilitates the transport of carbon dioxide.

White Blood Cells (WBCs)   also called leukocytes
Concentration   5 – 10 thousand / mm^3.
Size   White blood cells vary in diameter from 10 to 20 micrometers.
Function   The major function of white blood cells is to defend the body against pathogenic organisms (bacteria and viruses) and other foreign matter.
Types   The five types of white blood cells include :
   (1) Neutrophils (60 – 70% of total WBCs) Phagocytize pathogens.
   (2) Lymphocytes (20 – 25%) Produce antibodies and antimicrobial chemicals.
   (3) Monocytes (3 – 8%) Phagocytize pathogens.
   (4) Eosinophils (2 – 4%) Involved in defense against parasites and in the allergic response.
   (5) Basophils (0.5 – 1.0%) Secrete histamine.

Platelets   also called thrombocytes
Concentration   300 thousand / mm^3.
Size   Platelets have a diameter of 2 – 4 micrometers.
Function   Platelets are cell fragments that play crucial roles in blood clotting.

BLOOD COMPOSITION

Plasma

Serum

water
nutrients
wastes
hormones
antibodies
plasma proteins

Fibrinogen

function:
blood clotting

Cells

Platelets
(Thrombocytes)

300 thousand / mm^3
cell fragments formed from
megakaryocytes
function : blood clotting

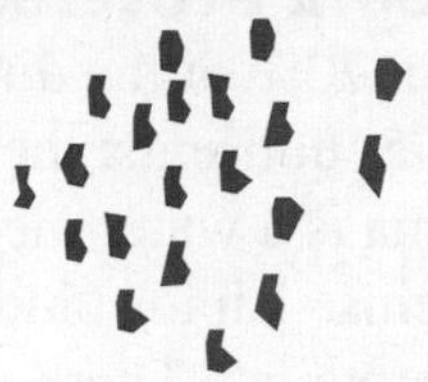

White Blood Cells
(Leukocytes)

5 – 10 thousand / mm^3

Red Blood Cells
(Erythrocytes)

5 – 6.5 million / mm^3

no nucleus   biconcave

Granulocytes
(Polymorphs)

granular cytoplasm;
lobed nucleus

Neutrophils
60 – 70 %

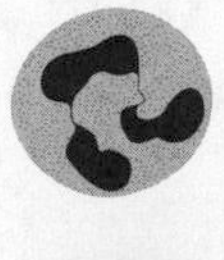

Eosinophils
2 – 4 %

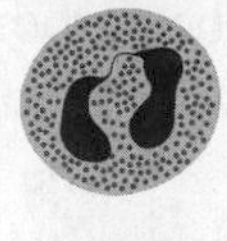

Basophils
0.5 – 1 %

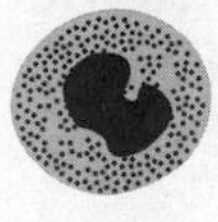

Agranulocytes

nongranular cytoplasm;
spherical or bean-shaped nucleus

Lymphocytes
20 – 25 %

Monocytes
3 – 8 %

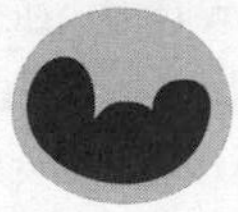

BLOOD / Plasma

Plasma   Plasma is the clear, straw-colored, liquid portion of the blood.
Serum   When fibrinogen and the other clotting factors are removed from plasma, the remaining liquid is called serum.

Water
Plasma is approximately 91.5% water and 8.5% (by weight) solutes. A complex mixture of organic and inorganic substances is dissolved in the water.

Plasma Proteins
About 70% of the dissolved substances in plasma are proteins. These plasma proteins are not used as nutrients; they perform various functions in the plasma and in the interstitial fluid. Since plasma is a water medium and lipids are insoluble in water, lipids must be bound to plasma proteins. Lipids bind to the hydrophobic portions of a protein molecule, forming water-soluble lipoproteins. There are three main types of plasma proteins : albumins, globulins, and coagulation factors.
  Albumins : maintain plasma osmotic pressure and blood volume; transport lipids.
  Alpha Globulins : transport lipids, copper, and thyroxine.
  Beta Globulins : transport lipids, iron, and heme.
  Gamma Globulins : (immunoglobulins) the circulating antibodies.
  Fibrinogen : precursor of fibrin (clot formation).
  Prothrombin : precursor of thrombin (clot formation).

Nonprotein Organic Components
About 20% of the dissolved substances are small organic molecules.
  Nutrients : amino acids, glucose, fatty acids, and glycerol.
  Wastes : urea, uric acid, creatine, creatinine, bilirubin, and ammonium salts.
      (All lipids are bound to plasma proteins to make them soluble in water.)

Inorganic Components
The remaining 10% of the dissolved substances are inorganic salts, buffers, and gases.

  Salts (Electrolytes)   The salts include : sodium chloride, calcium chloride, magnesium chloride, potassium chloride, sodium sulfate. Because these salts dissociate in water to form ions, they are called electrolytes.

  Buffers   Phosphates and bicarbonates are important buffers, absorbing or releasing hydrogen ions to maintain the normal pH level.

  Gases   Carbon dioxide, oxygen, and nitrogen. Most of the carbon dioxide transported by the blood is dissolved in the plasma; about 7% is in the form of carbon dioxide molecules and about 70% is in the form of the bicarbonate ion.   Only 3% of the oxygen transported by blood is dissolved in the plasma; the other 97% is combined with hemoglobin in the form of oxyhemoglobin. Nitrogen has no known function in the body.

PLASMA

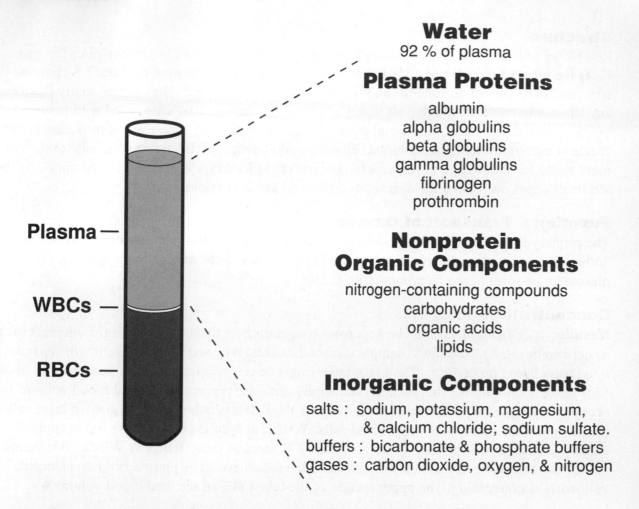

Plasma —

WBCs —

RBCs —

Water
92 % of plasma

Plasma Proteins
albumin
alpha globulins
beta globulins
gamma globulins
fibrinogen
prothrombin

Nonprotein Organic Components
nitrogen-containing compounds
carbohydrates
organic acids
lipids

Inorganic Components
salts : sodium, potassium, magnesium,
& calcium chloride; sodium sulfate.
buffers : bicarbonate & phosphate buffers
gases : carbon dioxide, oxygen, & nitrogen

Electrolyte Composition of Blood Plasma

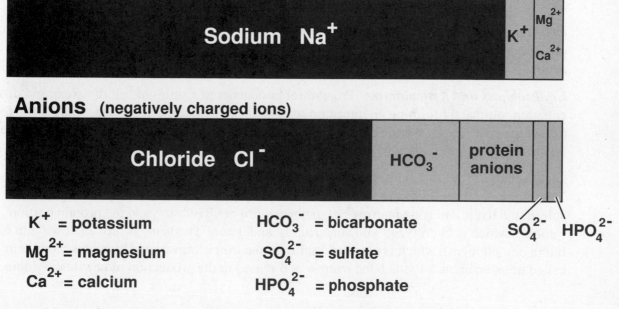

Cations (positively charged ions)

Sodium Na^+ K^+ Mg^{2+} Ca^{2+}

Anions (negatively charged ions)

Chloride Cl^- HCO_3^- protein anions SO_4^{2-} HPO_4^{2-}

K^+ = potassium HCO_3^- = bicarbonate

Mg^{2+} = magnesium SO_4^{2-} = sulfate

Ca^{2+} = calcium HPO_4^{2-} = phosphate

BLOOD / Red Blood Cells

Structure
Red blood cells (RBCs; also called erythrocytes) have the shape of a biconcave disc; this provides the greatest possible surface area for gas exchange. The diameter is about 7.5 micrometers, just small enough to squeeze through the lumen of a capillary. They are normally flexible and can easily be deformed to pass through narrow capillaries. RBCs are filled with hemoglobin, a protein that is used to transport oxygen and carbon dioxide. There are approximately 900 grams of hemoglobin in the red blood cells of an adult man. A RBC has no nucleus (this gives more space for the storage of hemoglobin). The ABO blood type of a RBC is determined by the terminal sugars on plasma membrane glycoproteins and glycolipids.

Function : Transport of Oxygen
The primary function of red blood cells is to transport oxygen from the lungs to the tissue cells. Although some carbon dioxide is transported by red blood cells, most is transported in the plasma in the form of the bicarbonate ion (HCO_3^-).

Concentration (hematocrit)
Hematocrit Drawn blood may be kept from coagulating by the addition of anticoagulants such as heparin or citrate. If a blood sample is placed in a test tube and centrifuged, it will separate into layers based on density. The lower layer (most dense) consists of RBCs and occupies about 45% of the total volume; this is called the hematocrit—the percentage of total blood volume occupied by red blood cells. Immediately above the RBCs is a thin white or grayish layer called the buffy coat; it consists of white blood cells (WBCs; also called leukocytes) and occupies about 1% of the total volume. There are about 700 times as many RBCs as WBCs. Above the WBCs is a fine layer of platelets not visible by the naked eye. The plasma is the translucent, yellowish viscous fluid in the upper portion of the tube (54% of the total blood volume).

Formation and Elimination
Erythropoiesis The formation of red blood cells (erythrocytes) occurs in the red bone marrow and is called erythropoiesis. During embryonic development blood cells arise from the yolk sac mesoderm, the liver, and spleen. During fetal development, when bone marrow has formed, the predominant tissue for blood cell production becomes the bone marrow.

Erythropoietin Erythropoietin is a hormone that stimulates stem cells in the red bone marrow to differentiate into proerythroblasts. About 85% of erythropoietin comes from the kidneys and about 15% from the liver. It is secreted in response to low plasma oxygen.

Erythroblasts and Reticulocytes Proerythroblasts undergo a series of cell divisions and differentiation, ultimately forming an immature red blood cell called a reticulocyte. During the formation of the reticulocyte hemoglobin is produced and the nucleus is expelled from the cell. Reticulocytes enter the circulation by penetrating the walls of the sinusoidal capillaries.

Destruction of RBCs Red blood cells have an average life span of 120 days. Every day about 200 billion red blood cells are produced and 200 billion are destroyed. Macrophages in the spleen, the liver, and bone marrow phagocytize worn out RBCs to yield the protein portion (globin), which is hydrolyzed into amino acids and heme. The heme is broken down into bilirubin (a bile pigment), which is excreted, and iron; the iron is transported by a plasma protein called transferrin back to the bone marrow and reused in the production of new hemoglobin.

RED BLOOD CELLS

Red Blood Cell (Erythrocyte)

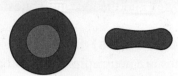

Hematocrit
Percent of RBCs by Volume

Plasma —

WBCs —

RBCs —
45 %

Hemoglobin Molecule
(schematic)

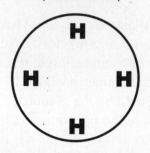

Each hemoglobin molecule contains 4 heme groups (H).

Heme Group

Each heme group contains 1 iron atom which binds 1 oxygen molecule

BLOOD / White Blood Cells

The function of white blood cells (leukocytes) is to defend the body against foreign materials: pathogenic microorganisms (bacteria and viruses), parasitic worms, toxins, tumors, and organ transplants. There are 5 basic types of white blood cells : neutrophils, eosinophils, basophils, lymphocytes, and monocytes. Based on the shape of their nucleus and the type of granules in their cytoplasm, they are divided into two groups: the granulocytes and the agranulocytes.

GRANULOCYTES (also called Granular Leukocytes)

Neutrophils   60 – 70% of the circulating leukocytes are neutrophils; the cell diameter is between 12 and 15 micrometers. The nucleus usually consists of 3 lobes linked by fine threads of chromatin. They contain two types of granules : Specific granules are membrane-bound vesicles that contain chemicals that kill bacteria; they have a diameter of 0.1 micrometer, barely visible in the light microscope. Azurophilic granules contain a large variety of enzymes that digest bacteria after they are dead, breaking them down into basic chemicals that can be used by nearby cells as nutrients; they are larger, having a diameter of 0.5 micrometer.

Phagocytosis   Neutrophils kill bacteria by phagocytosis. They surround a bacterium with pseudopodia, forming a vacuole, called a phagosome. Granules fuse with the phagosome and release their chemicals, which kill and digest the bacterium.

Eosinophils   2 – 4% of the circulating leukocytes; cell diameter is 12 – 15 micrometers. An eosinophil has a bilobed nucleus and large granules (0.5 – 1.5 micrometers). An increase in the number of eosinophils is associated with parasitic worm infections and allergic reactions.

Basophils   0.5 – 1.0% of the circulating leukocytes; cell diameter is 12 – 15 micrometers. A basophil has an irregular-lobed nucleus that is usually obscured by the granules. The granules contain *heparin* and *histamine*. They are similar to mast cells found in connective tissues.

AGRANULOCYTES   (also called Agranular Leukocytes)

Lymphocytes   20 – 25% of the circulating leukocytes. Lymphocytes are a family of cells, not one particular cell type. Most lymphocytes are small (6 – 8 micrometers) with a spherical nucleus that occupies most of the cell; there are also medium and large lymphocytes with diameters up to 18 micrometers. They are produced in the bone marrow, differentiated in the bone marrow and thymus, and reside in the spleen, lymph nodes, tonsils, and other lymphoid tissues.

B Cells   Lymphocytes that differentiate in the bone marrow are called B cells (also called B lymphocytes). About 15% of the circulating lymphocytes are B cells. There are thousands of different types of B cells, each primed to respond to only one type of antigen. When B cells come into contact with their specific antigen, they are converted into plasma cells. Plasma cells then produce antibodies for that particular antigen.

T Cells   Lymphocytes that differentiate in the thymus are called T cells (also called T lymphocytes). About 80% of the circulating lymphocytes are T cells (the remaining 5% of T cells are called Null cells, and are presumed to be stem cells). *Helper T cells* and *supressor T cells* stimulate and inhibit the activites of other lymphocytes; *cytotoxic T cells* directly kill tumor cells, virus-infected cells, and foreign tissue grafts by making holes in their membranes; other T cells release chemicals that stimulate macrophages to migrate toward infection sites.

Monocytes   3 – 8% of circulating leukocytes; cell diameter 12 – 20 micrometers. The nucleus is oval, horseshoe-shaped, or kidney-shaped. After crossing capillary walls and entering tissue spaces monocytes differentiate into macrophages (large phagocytes). They play important roles in the recognition and interaction of leukocytes with antigens.

WHITE BLOOD CELLS

Neutrophil
60 – 70 % of WBCs

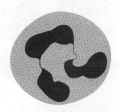

Phagocytize (eat) bacteria
(acute infections; first defense)

Eosinophil
2 – 4 % of WBCs

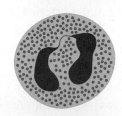

Defense mechanism
for parasitic worms

Basophil
0.5 – 1 % of WBCs

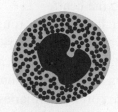

Secrete histamine;
enter tissue spaces
and become mast cells

Lymphocyte
20 – 25 % of WBCs

Specialize in lymphatic tissues:
B cells produce antibodies;
T cells secrete lysing enzymes

Monocyte
3 – 8 % of WBCs

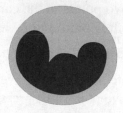

Phagocytize (eat) bacteria
(chronic infections);
enter tissue spaces
and become macrophages

Platelets
(WBC fragments)

Involved in the blood
clotting mechanism

BLOOD / Hemodynamics

The principles that govern the flow of any fluid (liquid or gas) through a tube apply to blood flowing through blood vessels and air flowing through the airways of the lungs. Fluids flow from regions of higher to lower pressure; resistance, caused by friction between the molecules of the fluid and the walls of the tube, reduces the flow.

VELOCITY OF BLOOD FLOW
Total Cross–Sectional Area
The velocity of blood flow is inversely related to the total cross-sectional area of the blood vessels. The aorta is the largest artery, but it branches into many arteries that have a combined cross-sectional area that is many times that of the aorta. The same 5 liters of blood that are pumped into the aorta during each cardiac cycle, must pass through all of the capillaries during the same minute. Because there are a vast number of capillaries, their total cross-sectional area is hundreds of times greater than that of the aorta. So the blood velocity decreases from about 40 cm/sec to 0.1 cm/sec.

As blood returns to the heart, the total cross-sectional area of the veins gradually decreases and the blood velocity increases. In a resting adult, it takes a red blood cell about one minute to travel from the heart, through the blood vessels, and back to the heart.

Aorta When blood leaves the left ventricle it passes through a single tube, the aorta, with a cross-sectional area of about 3 cm^2, and its average velocity is 40 cm/sec.

Arteries and Arterioles Because the total cross-sectional area of the arteries and arterioles is greater than that of the aorta, the velocity decreases as it flows through these vessels.

Capillaries The total cross-sectional area of the capillaries is about 5000 cm^2 and the velocity of blood flow is about 0.1cm/sec.

Veins and Venules Because the total cross-sectional area of the veins and venules is less than that of the capillaries, the velocity increases as it flows back to the heart.

Venae Cavae The combined cross-sectional area of the two venae cavae is about 14 cm^2 and the velocity of blood flow is 5 to 20 cm/sec.

VOLUME OF BLOOD FLOW
The volume of blood flow between any two points in the cardiovascular system is directly proportional to the pressure difference between the points and inversely proportional to the resistance.

Flow = Pressure Gradient / Resistance

Pressure Gradient It is not the absolute pressure at a given point that determines the blood flow; it is the difference in pressures between two points (the pressure gradient). When considering blood flow through the systemic circulation from the aorta to the right atrium, the relevant pressures are the mean arterial blood pressure and the pressure in the right atrium. At rest the mean (average) arterial blood pressure (MABP) is about 93 mm Hg; the blood pressure in the right atrium is close to 0 mm Hg.

Resistance Resistance refers to the opposition to flow that results from friction between blood and the walls of the blood vessels. It cannot be directly measured; it can be calculated from the directly measured flow and pressure gradient. Resistance is directly proportional to the viscosity (thickness) of the blood and the length of the blood vessel; it is inversely proportional to the fourth power of the lumen diameter. Since the viscosity of blood and the length of blood vessels do not change under normal circumstances, the resistance to blood flow is determined by the diameter of the blood vessels. And, since arterioles are the blood vessels that have the greatest capacity for change in diameter, they determine the resistance. A very small change in the diameter of an arteriole causes a significant change in the resistance : doubling the diameter decreases the resistance 16-fold.

HEMODYNAMICS

VELOCITY OF BLOOD FLOW
Relationship Between Velocity and Total Cross–Sectional Area
Velocity of blood flow varies inversely with
the total cross-sectional area of the vessels.

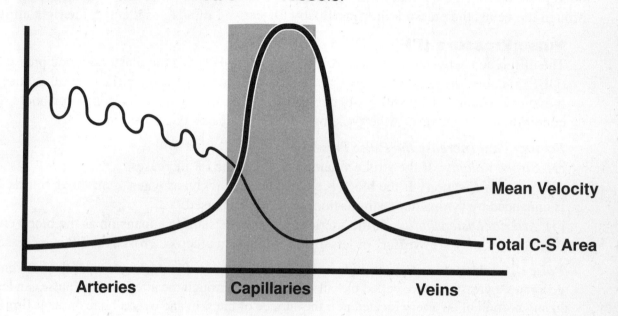

VOLUME OF BLOOD FLOW

$$\text{Flow} = \frac{\text{Pressure Gradient}}{\text{Resistance}} \qquad F = \frac{\Delta P}{R}$$

$$\Delta P = \text{Mean Arterial Pressure} - \text{Right Atrial Pressure}$$

$$R = \frac{\text{Viscosity of Blood} \quad X \quad \text{Length of Tube}}{(\text{Diameter of Lumen})^4}$$

SYSTEMIC CIRCULATION

In the arteries and arterioles the blood pressure rises and falls with each heartbeat, causing a pulsing (irregular) flow of blood. Because of the low resistance offered by the large-diameter arteries, the pressures remain relatively constant as blood passes through these vessels. The high resistance of the arterioles causes a sharp drop in blood pressure from about 85 to 35 mm Hg. As blood passes through a capillary the pressure drops from 35 to 16 mm Hg. While passing through the veins, the pressure drops gradually to nearly 0 mm Hg as it enters the right atrium.

Pulse Pressure (PP)   PP = SBP – DBP

The difference between the systolic blood pressure (SBP) and the diastolic blood pressure (DBP) is called the pulse pressure (PP). When the arterial pressure is 120 / 80, the pulse pressure is equal to 120 – 80 = 40 mm Hg. This pressure provides information about the condition of the arteries. Atherosclerosis greatly increases pulse pressure.

Factors That Increase the Pulse Pressure
(1) Stroke Volume   If the stroke volume increases, the PP increases.
(2) Speed of Ejection   If the blood is ejected more quickly, as when ventricular contractility is enhanced by sympathetic stimulation, the PP is increased.
(3) Arterial Distensibility   If the arteries are more resistant to expansion as the blood enters them (i.e., if they are "stiffer" or less distensible), as in atherosclerosis, the PP is increased.

Pulse   The alternate expansion and recoil of elastic arteries after each systole of the left ventricle generates a pressure wave called the pulse that travels through the arteries. The pulse can be felt in any portion of an artery located near the surface of the skin and over a bone or other firm surface. The radial artery at the wrist is most commonly used to feel the pulse.

Mean Arterial Blood Pressure (MABP)   MABP = DBP + 1/3 PP

The mean arterial blood pressure is important because it is the pressure driving blood into the tissues throughout the cardiac cycle. The mean pressure in the systemic arteries is about 93 mm Hg and the pressure in the right atrium is close to 0 mm Hg, so the pressure gradient forcing blood through the systemic system is about 93 mm Hg.

The arterial pressure is constantly changing throughout the cardiac cycle. The MABP is not merely the value halfway between systolic and diastolic pressure. Since diastole lasts longer than systole, the mean pressure is not a simple average; it is a function of time. It is approximately equal to the diastolic pressure plus 1/3 of the pulse pressure. It is closely regulated by the basic cardiovascular control mechanisms.

PULMONARY CIRCULATION

Although the cardiac output is identical for the left and right ventricles, the blood pressures in the pulmonary and systemic systems are very different. The pulmonary vascular system is an elastic (distensible) low-pressure system. The walls of the vessels are thin and stretchy, offering little resistance to flow.

The mean pressure in the pulmonary arteries is only 15 mm Hg (systolic : 24 mm Hg; diastolic : 9 mm Hg). During diastole, the pressure in the left atrium is about 8 mm Hg, so the pressure gradient forcing blood from the lungs back to the heart is only about 7 mm Hg.

PRESSURE CHANGES IN THE SYSTEMIC CIRCULATION

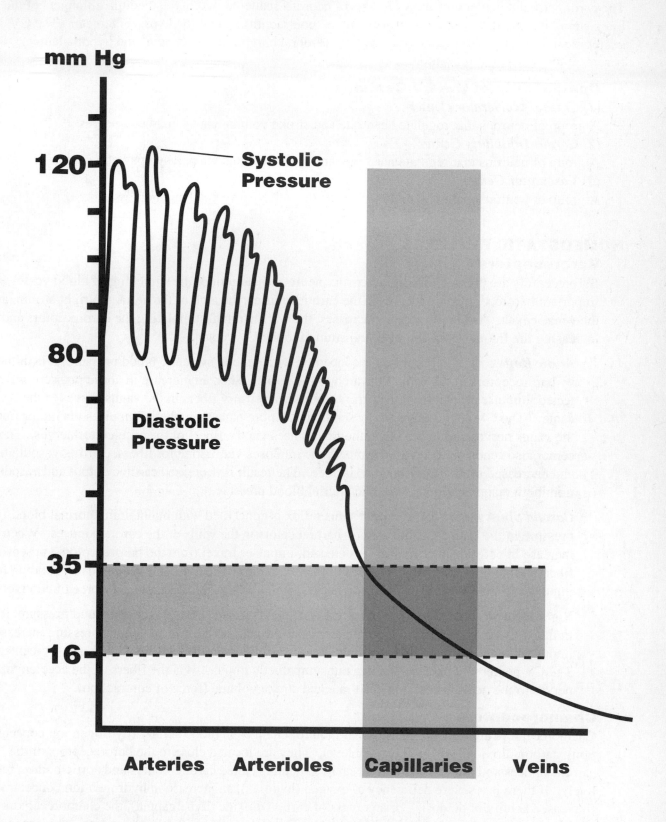

BLOOD / Blood Pressure : Neural Regulation

CARDIOVASCULAR CENTER (CV Center)

The cardiovascular center consists of groups of neurons scattered within the medulla oblongata of the brain stem. It regulates heart rate, stroke volume (contractility), and blood vessel diameter. The CV center receives input from higher brain centers (cerebral cortex, limbic system, and hypothalamus), baroreceptors, and chemoreceptors.

Components of the CV Center

(1) Cardio-Accelerator Center
A group of neurons that regulate heart rate and stroke volume via sympathetic nerves.
(2) Cardio-Inhibitory Center
A group of neurons that regulate heart rate and stroke volume via parasympathetic nerves.
(3) Vasomotor Center
A group of neurons that regulate blood vessel diameter via sympathetic nerves.

HOMEOSTATIC REFLEXES

Baroreceptors

Baroreceptors are pressure-sensitive sensory neurons that monitor the stretching of blood vessel walls. Important baroreceptors are located in the carotid sinuses, the arch of the aorta, the right atrium, and the venae cavae. As blood pressure increases, the walls stretch, stimulating the baroreceptors and increasing the frequency of impulses transmitted to the CV center.

Aortic Reflex   The aortic reflex is concerned with general systemic blood pressure; it is initiated by baroreceptors in the wall of the arch of the aorta. When an increase in aortic pressure is detected, impulses travel from the baroreceptors via sensory fibers in the vagus nerves to the CV center. The CV center responds by sending out more parasympathetic impulses via motor fibers of the vagus nerves and fewer sympathetic impulses via the fibers of the accelerator nerves. The CV center also sends out decreased sympathetic impulses via vasomotor fibers, causing vasodilation and decreased systemic vascular resistance. The result is decreased cardiac output and vasodilation; both responses lower systemic arterial blood pressure.

Carotid Sinus Reflex   The carotid sinus reflex is concerned with maintaining normal blood pressure in the brain; it is initiated by baroreceptors in the walls of the carotid sinuses. When an increase in carotid sinus pressure is detected, impulses travel from the baroreceptors via sensory fibers in the glossopharyngeal nerves to the CV center. The CV center responds by sending fewer impulses to the heart via sympathetic nerves, which decreases heart rate and force of contraction.

Right Heart Reflex   The right heart reflex responds to increases in venous blood pressure; it is initiated by baroreceptors in the right atrium and venae cavae. When venous pressure increases, impulses travel from the baroreceptors via sensory fibers in the vagus nerves to the CV center. The CV center responds by sending out sympathetic impulses via the fibers of the accelerator nerves to the heart, increasing heart rate and stroke volume (force of contraction).

Chemoreceptors

Chemoreceptors are sensory neurons that monitor changes in blood acidity (hydrogen ion concentration), carbon dioxide level, and oxygen level. They are located close to the baroreceptors of the carotid sinuses and arch of the aorta in small structures called carotid bodies and aortic bodies, respectively. If there is a severe deficiency of oxygen (hypoxia), an increase in hydrogen ion concentration (increased acidity or acidosis), or an excess of carbon dioxide (hypercapnia), the chemoreceptors are stimulated and send impulses to the CV center. The CV center responds by sending impulses to the heart via sympathetic nerves, which increase heart rate and force of contraction.

BLOOD PRESSURE : Neural Regulation

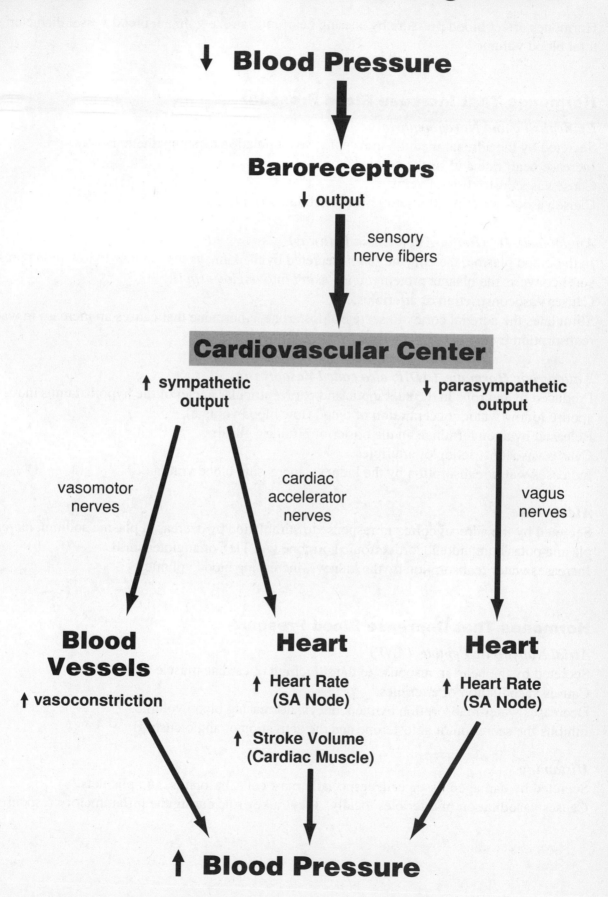

↓ **Blood Pressure**

Baroreceptors

↓ output

sensory
nerve fibers

Cardiovascular Center

↑ sympathetic
output

↓ parasympathetic
output

vasomotor
nerves

cardiac
accelerator
nerves

vagus
nerves

**Blood
Vessels**

↑ vasoconstriction

Heart

↑ Heart Rate
(SA Node)

↑ Stroke Volume
(Cardiac Muscle)

Heart

↑ Heart Rate
(SA Node)

↑ **Blood Pressure**

BLOOD / Blood Pressure : Hormonal Regulation

Hormones affect blood pressure by altering heart rate, stroke volume, blood vessel diameter, or total blood volume.

Hormones That Increase Blood Pressure

Epinephrine and Norepinephrine
Secreted by the adrenal medulla in response to stimulation by sympathetic nerves.
Increase heart rate and stroke volume (contractility).
Cause vasoconstriction of veins.
Cause vasoconstriction of arterioles of the abdomen and skin.

Angiotensin II   (Renin-Angiotensin Pathway)
In the blood plasma, the enzyme *renin* (secreted by the kidneys in response to low blood pressure) converts the plasma protein *angiotensin I* into *angiotensin II*.
Causes vasoconstriction of arterioles.
Stimulates the adrenal cortex to secrete aldosterone, a hormone that causes an increase in water reabsorption by the kidneys, increasing blood volume.

Antidiuretic Hormone (ADH; also called Vasopressin)
Produced by neurons in the supraoptic and paraventricular nuclei of the hypothalamus in response to low water concentration of blood (low blood volume).
Released by axon terminals in the posterior pituitary gland.
Causes vasoconstriction of arterioles.
Increases water reabsorption by the kidneys, increasing blood volume.

Aldosterone
Secreted by the adrenal cortex in response to stimulation by decreased plasma sodium, increased plasma potassium, adrenocorticotropic hormone (ACTH), or angiotensin II.
Increases water reabsorption by the kidneys, increasing blood volume.

Hormones That Decrease Blood Pressure

Atrial Natriuretic Peptide (ANP)
Secreted by the heart in response to the stretching of cardiac muscle fibers.
Causes vasodilation of arterioles.
Decreases water reabsorption by the kidneys, decreasing blood volume.
Inhibits the secretion of aldosterone and the activation of angiotensin II.

Histamine
Secreted by damaged tissue cells; especially mast cells, basophils, and platelets.
Causes vasodilation of arterioles locally. Plays a key role during the inflammatory response.

BLOOD PRESSURE : Hormonal Regulation

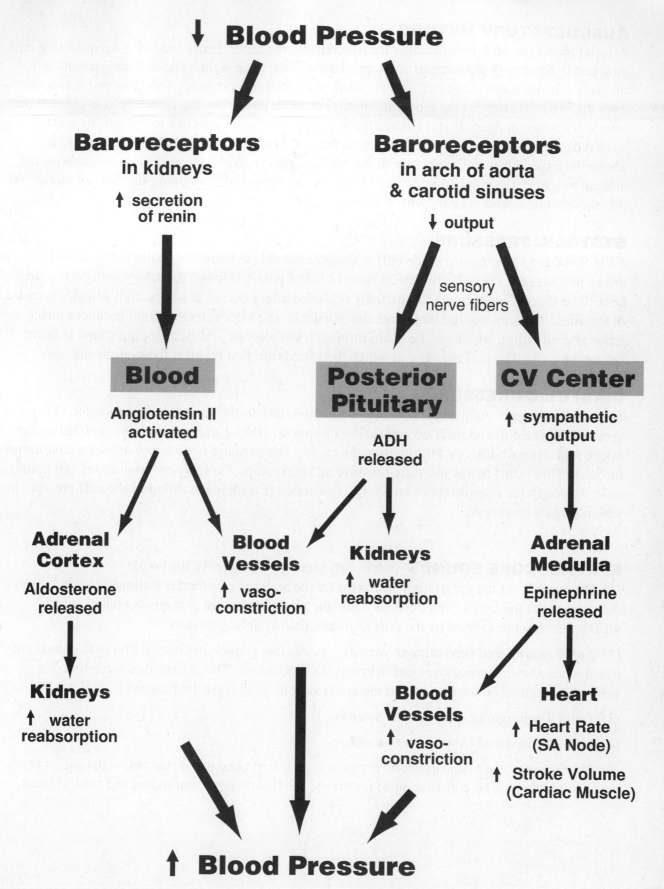

↓ **Blood Pressure**

Baroreceptors
in kidneys

↑ secretion
of renin

Baroreceptors
in arch of aorta
& carotid sinuses

↓ output

sensory
nerve fibers

Blood

Angiotensin II
activated

**Posterior
Pituitary**

ADH
released

CV Center

↑ sympathetic
output

**Adrenal
Cortex**

Aldosterone
released

**Blood
Vessels**

↑ vaso-
constriction

Kidneys

↑ water
reabsorption

**Adrenal
Medulla**

Epinephrine
released

Kidneys

↑ water
reabsorption

**Blood
Vessels**

↑ vaso-
constriction

Heart

↑ Heart Rate
(SA Node)

↑ Stroke Volume
(Cardiac Muscle)

↑ **Blood Pressure**

BLOOD / Blood Pressure : Measurement

AUSCULTATORY METHOD

Arterial blood pressure is commonly measured using the auscultatory method. An inflatable cuff attached to a mercury manometer is wrapped around the upper arm. The mercury manometer measures the pressure in the cuff and is called a sphygmomanometer. A stethoscope is placed over the brachial artery at the elbow to monitor changes caused by the flow of blood through the artery. Pressure in the cuff is regulated by a rubber bulb that is attached to the cuff by a tube.

To determine the arterial blood pressure, the cuff is rapidly inflated until the pressure is above the expected systolic pressure in the brachial artery. When the cuff pressure is above the arterial pressure, the brachial artery will be occluded (closed off), stopping the flow of blood. At this moment no sound is heard with the stethoscope.

SYSTOLIC PRESSURE

First Sounds   The pressure in the cuff is slowly lowered. When the systolic pressure in the artery just exceeds the cuff pressure, a spurt of blood passes through the artery with each heartbeat. The blood flow through the partially occluded artery occurs at a very high velocity because of the small opening and the large pressure gradient. The high-velocity blood produces turbulence and vibration, which can be heard through a stethoscope. Also, a tapping sound is heard below the cuff. The cuff pressure at which the sounds are first heard is the systolic pressure.

DIASTOLIC PRESSURE

Sounds Disappear   As the cuff pressure is lowered further, the sounds become louder. Then the sounds become dull and muffled and finally disappear. The sounds are dull and muffled as the artery remains partially open throughout the cycle. The partially open artery allows a continuous turbulent flow. Just below diastolic pressure all sound stops; flow is now continuous and nonturbulent through the completely open artery. Diastolic pressure is identified as the cuff pressure at which sounds disappear.

STETHOSCOPE SOUNDS   (while cuff pressure is gradually lowered)

(1) No Sound   At the initial high cuff pressure the artery is completely flattened (occluded) by the pressure of the cuff. Even during systole the artery in the arm remains occluded, which means the pressure exerted by the cuff is greater than systolic pressure.

(2) Soft Tapping and Intermittent Sounds   *(just below systolic pressure)*   The first sounds are heard when the cuff pressure is just below systolic pressure. This means that some blood is getting through when the pressure in the artery is at its peak (systolic pressure).

(3) Loud Tapping and Intermittent Sounds

(4) Low Muffled and Continuous Sounds

(5) No Sound   *(just below diastolic pressure)*   This cuff pressure is just below diastolic pressure. Since there is no constriction of the artery, the flow is now continuous and nonturbulent.

MEASUREMENT OF BLOOD PRESSURE

Sphygmomanometer

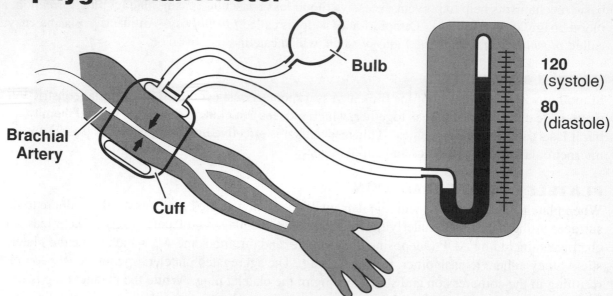

Bulb

Brachial Artery

Cuff

120 (systole)

80 (diastole)

Location of Stethoscope for Valve Sounds

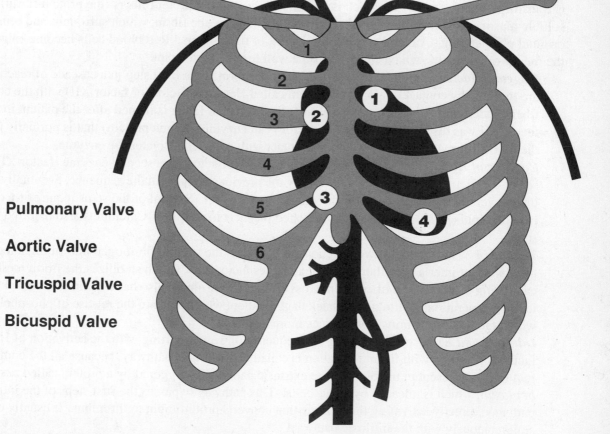

1 Pulmonary Valve

2 Aortic Valve

3 Tricuspid Valve

4 Bicuspid Valve

BLOOD / Hemostasis

The term *hemostasis* means to stop the flow of blood. When a small blood vessel is ruptured, three basic mechanisms help to prevent excessive blood loss : vascular spasm, platelet plug formation, and blood coagulation (clotting). Dissolution of a clot is called *fibrinolysis*. An inactive plasma enzyme called *plasminogen* is converted into *plasmin*, which can dissolve the clot.

VASCULAR SPASM

Smooth muscles in the wall of the broken vessel spontaneously contract. This initial constriction presses the endothelial surfaces together, which induces a stickiness that tends to hold them together, but it lasts for only a few minutes. This mechanism is effective only in the smallest vessels of the microcirculation (metarterioles and capillaries).

PLATELET PLUG FORMATION

When platelets make contact with the damaged inner lining of the blood vessel, they adhere to the surface. Adherence to the underlying connective tissue collagen molecules triggers the release of chemicals, including ADP (adenosine diphosphate) and thromboxane A2, which make the platelets sticky; they adhere to each other, forming a plug. The aggregated platelets spontaneously contract, resulting in the compression and strengthening of the platelet plug. While the platelet plug is forming, thromboxane A2 and other chemicals released by the platelets stimulate vasoconstriction in nearby vessels, decreasing blood flow to the damaged vessel. The most effective hemostatic mechanism is the formation of a blood clot, which involves a complex series of chemical reactions.

BLOOD COAGULATION (blood clot formation)

Coagulation is the transformation of a liquid into a semisolid or solid mass. In blood coagulation, plasma is transformed into a solid gel, which is composed of a mass of protein fibers (the protein fibrin). The soluble plasma protein fibrinogen is converted into the insolube fibrin, which surrounds and reinforces the original platelet plug. A blood clot is a meshwork of fibrin fibers. Red blood cells become entangled in the meshwork of fibers, which strengthens the wall formed by the clot.

Hageman factor (factor XII)   The formation of fibrin is the final step in a cascade of reactions that are initiated by contact of a plasma protein called Hageman factor (or factor XII) with the collagen fibers underlying the damaged vessel surface. Hageman factor is named after the patient in whom factor XII was discovered. Hageman factor is an enzyme (plasma protein) that is normally present in the blood plasma in an inactive form. Contact with collagen activates the enzyme.

Cascade of Reactions   The activated Hageman factor activates a second enzyme (factor XI). A series of inactive enzymes are activated by the previous enzyme in the sequence, eventually causing the conversion of the inactive prothrombin into thrombin. Several of the steps require as a cofactor a phospholipid (PF3) secreted by the activated platelets in the plug. Calcium is also required for certain steps.

Thrombin   Thrombin has two functions: It converts the soluble fibrinogen into fibrin, a loose meshwork of interlacing fibers. And it activates factor XIII, which stabilizes the fibrin meshwork by catalyzing the formation of covalent cross-linkages. Thrombin also has a positive feedback effect on its own generation: it stimulates platelet aggregation, which leads to the release of phospholipid, which facilitates reactions that produce more thrombin.

Intrinsic and Extrinsic Pathways   The sequence of events starting with the activation of Hageman factor and ending with fibrin formation is called the instrinsic pathway, because all the components required are present in the blood. The extrinsic pathway is triggered by a protein called *tissue thromboplastin*, which is released by tissue cells. This pathway bypasses the first steps of the intrinsic pathway, directly activating the enzyme that converts prothrombin to thrombin. It usually occurs simultaneously with the intrinsic pathway.

BLOOD CLOT FORMATION

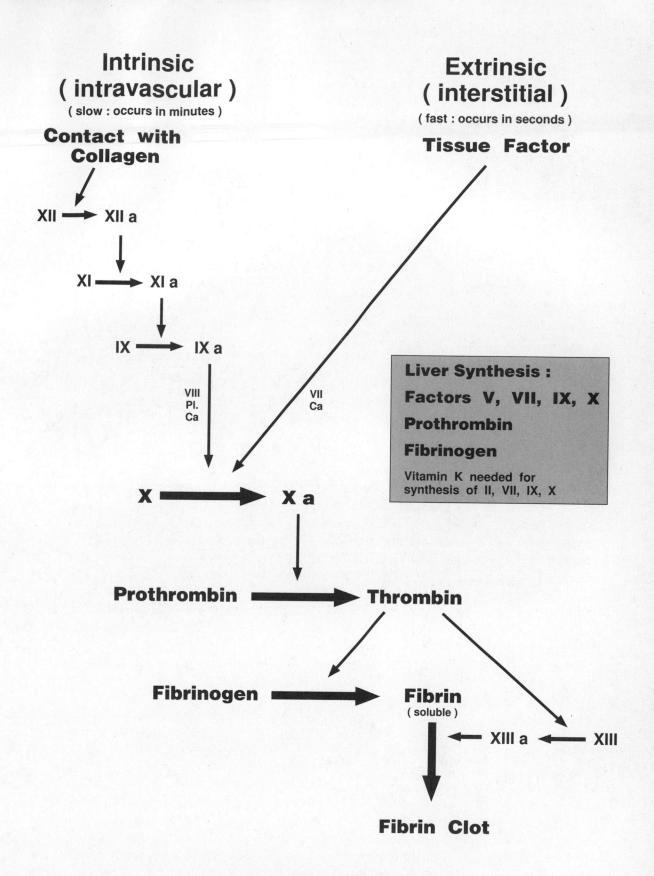

Intrinsic
(intravascular)
(slow : occurs in minutes)

Contact with
Collagen

XII → XII a

XI → XI a

IX → IX a

VIII
Pl.
Ca

Extrinsic
(interstitial)
(fast : occurs in seconds)

Tissue Factor

VII
Ca

X → X a

Liver Synthesis :
Factors V, VII, IX, X
Prothrombin
Fibrinogen
Vitamin K needed for
synthesis of II, VII, IX, X

Prothrombin → Thrombin

Fibrinogen → Fibrin
(soluble)

XIII a ← XIII

Fibrin Clot

Part II : Self-Testing Exercises

Unlabeled illustrations from Part I

CARDIOVASCULAR SYSTEM OVERVIEW

_____ Circulation : gray shading
_____ Circulation : white

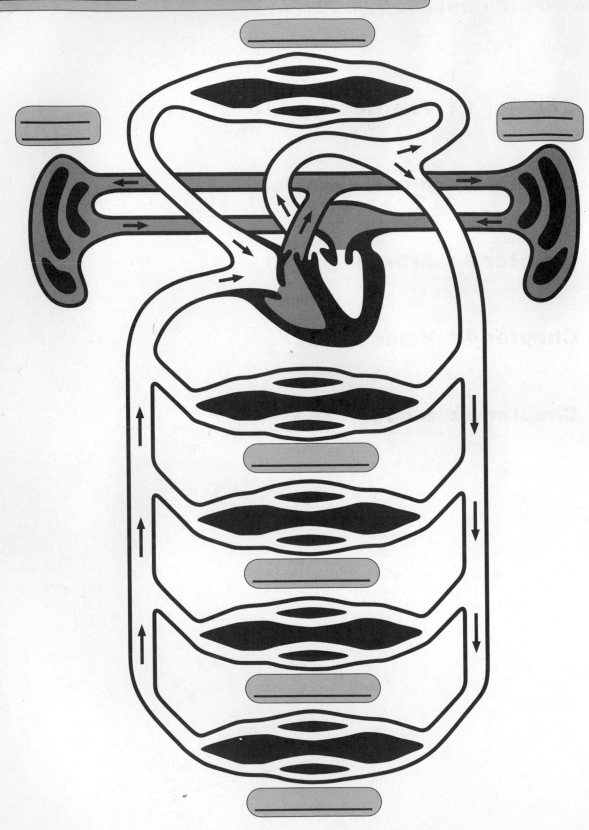

HEART ANATOMY
Superficial Anterior View

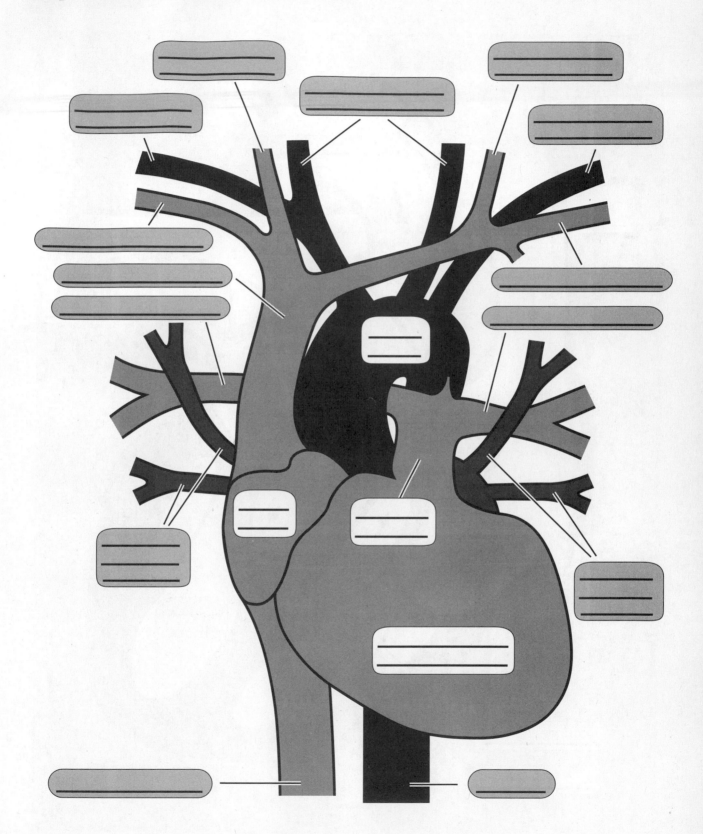

HEART ANATOMY
Chambers and Valves

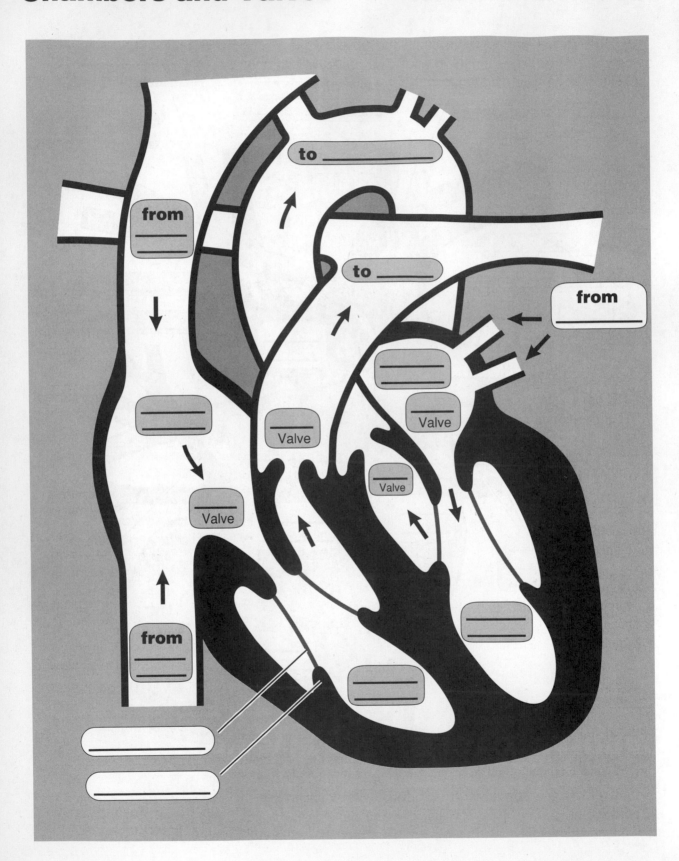

TISSUES
Cardiac Muscle

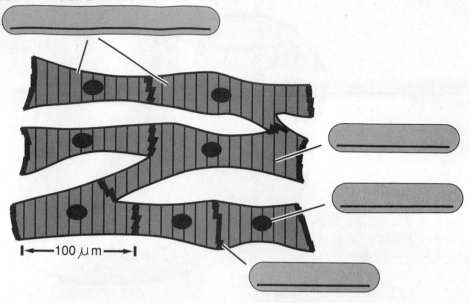

|←—100 μm—→|

Pericardium and Heart Wall

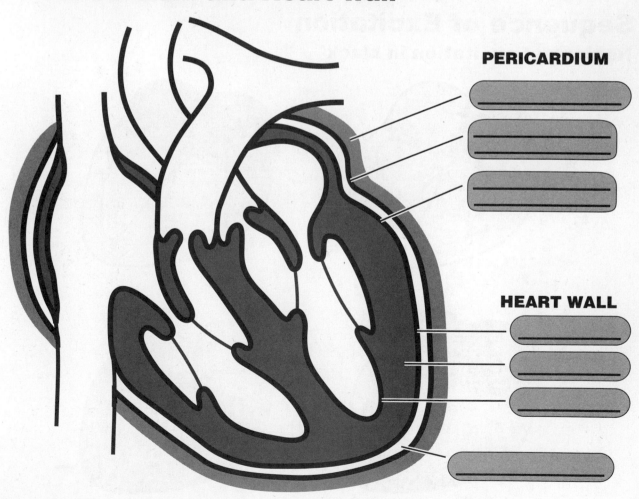

PERICARDIUM

HEART WALL

CONDUCTION SYSTEM

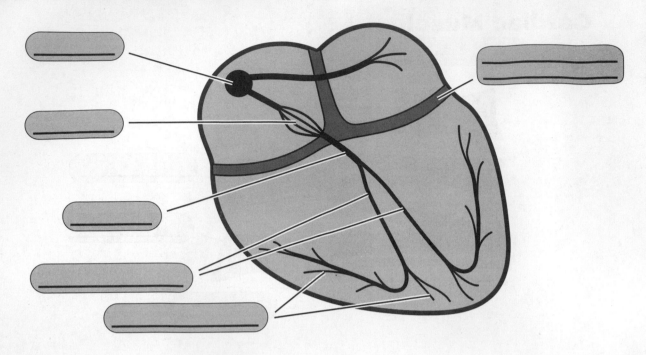

Sequence of Excitation
Regions of excitation in black

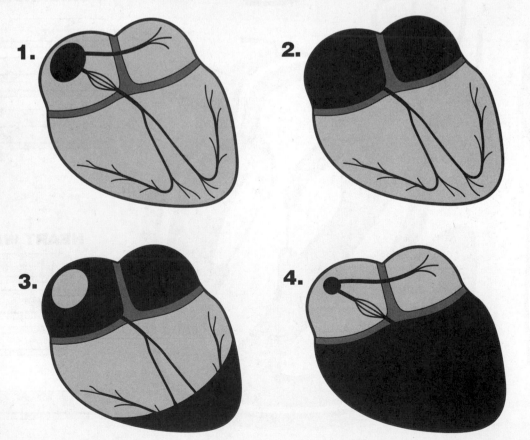

1.

2.

3.

4.

120

ACTION POTENTIALS
Cardiac Muscle compared to Skeletal Muscle

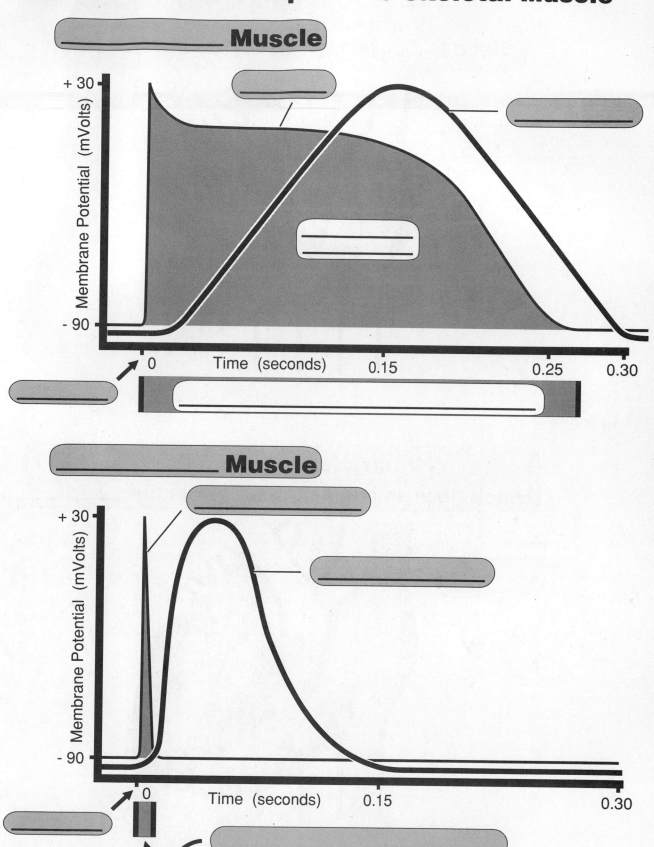

121

SYSTOLE AND DIASTOLE

Ventricles _____
Blood is ejected into the _____.

_____

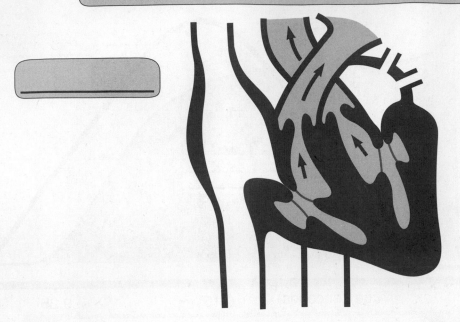

Ventricles _____
Blood flows into the _____ from the _____.

_____

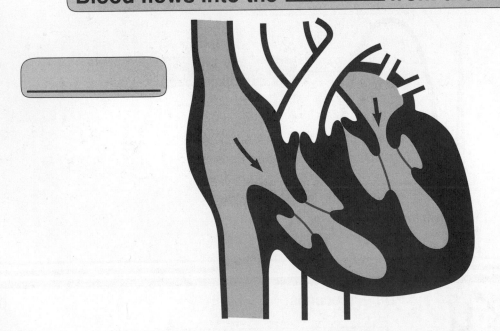

CARDIAC CYCLE : The Five Phases

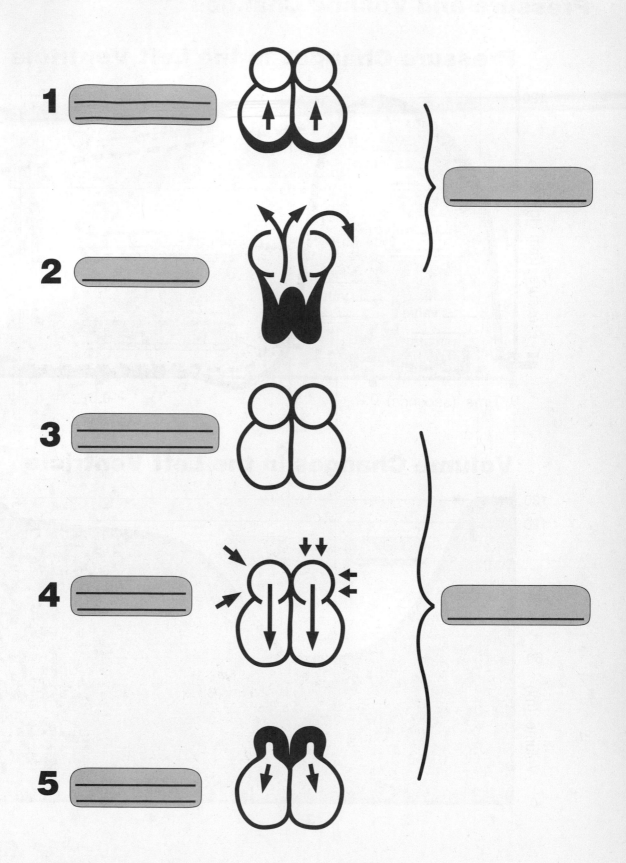

CARDIAC CYCLE
Pressure and Volume Changes

Pressure Changes in the Left Ventricle

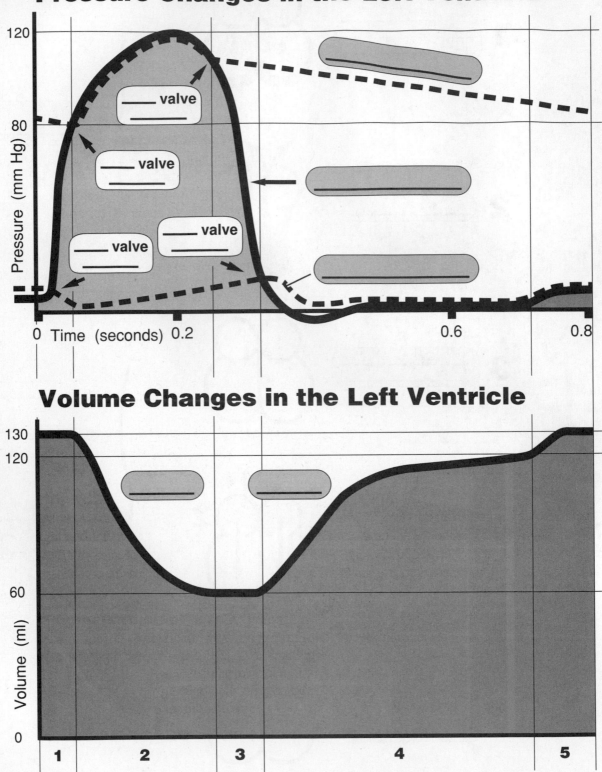

CARDIAC CYCLE : Summary

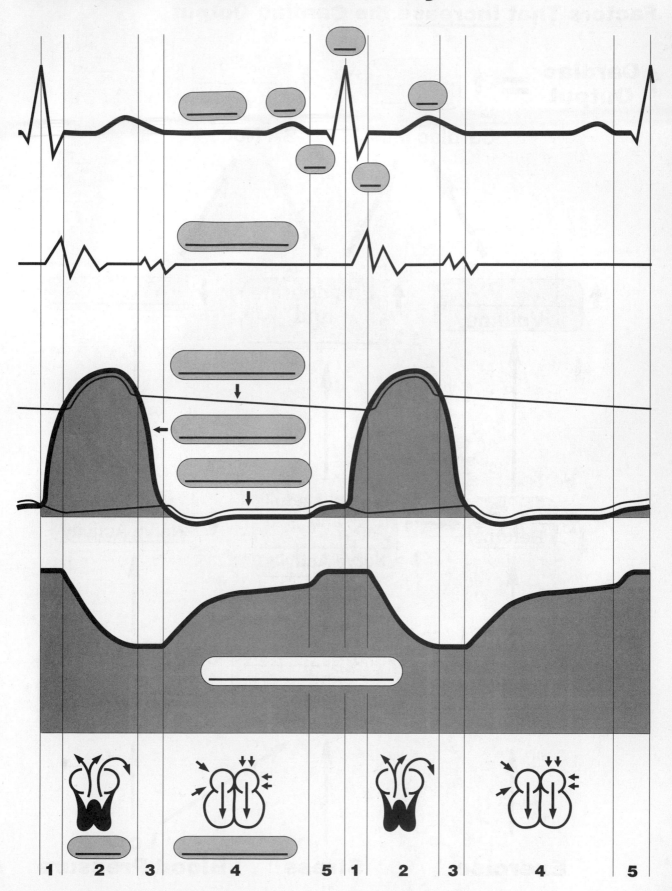

CARDIAC OUTPUT
Factors That <u>Increase</u> the Cardiac Output

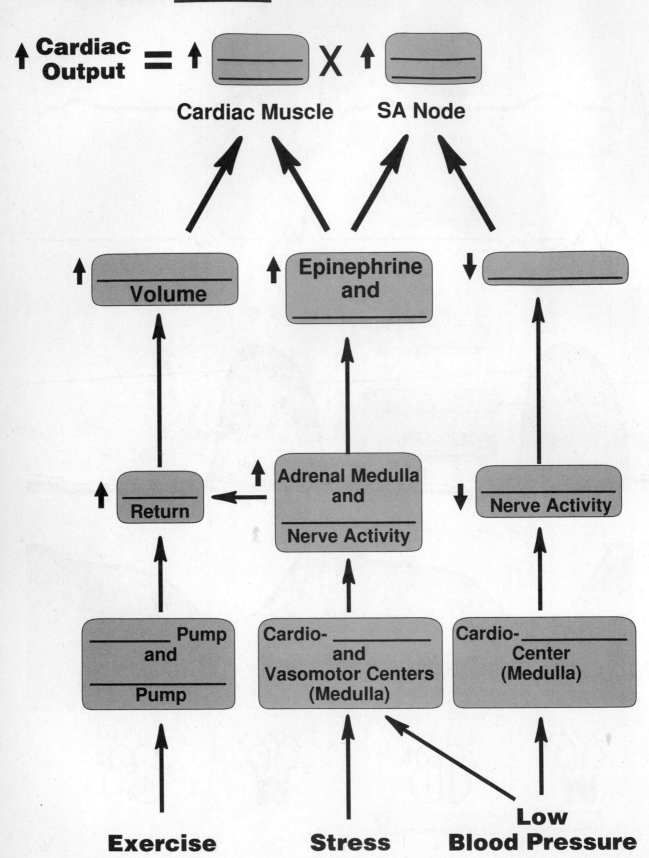

↑ Cardiac Output = ↑ ⬚ X ↑ ⬚

Cardiac Muscle   SA Node

↑ _____ Volume

↑ Epinephrine and _____

↓ _____

↑ _____ Return

↑ Adrenal Medulla and _____ Nerve Activity

↓ _____ Nerve Activity

_____ Pump and _____ Pump

Cardio-_____ and Vasomotor Centers (Medulla)

Cardio-_____ Center (Medulla)

Exercise   Stress   Low Blood Pressure

CARDIAC OUTPUT
Effect of Exercise on CO and Blood Distribution

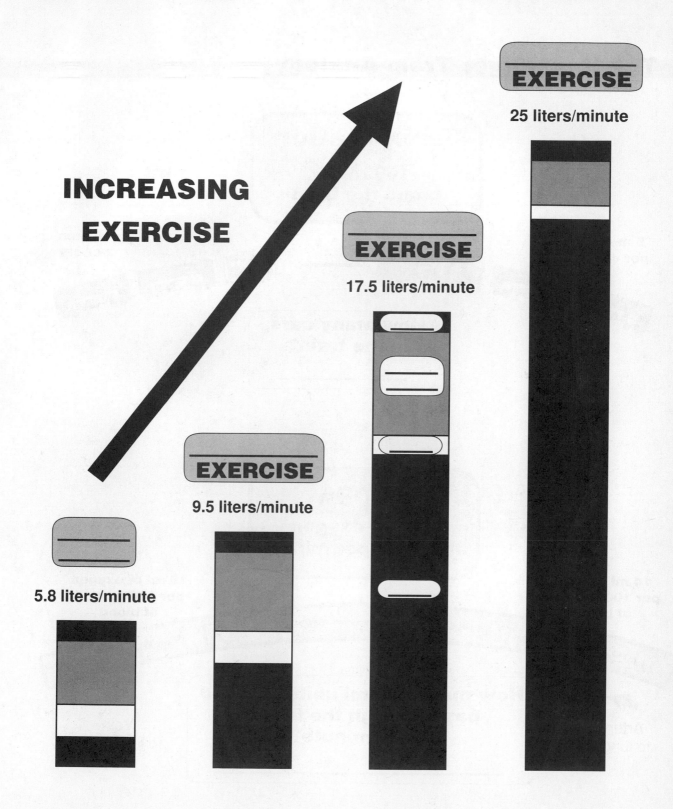

INCREASING EXERCISE

EXERCISE
25 liters/minute

EXERCISE
17.5 liters/minute

EXERCISE
9.5 liters/minute

EXERCISE
5.8 liters/minute

CARDIAC OUTPUT
Measured by the Fick Method

The Passenger Train Analogy

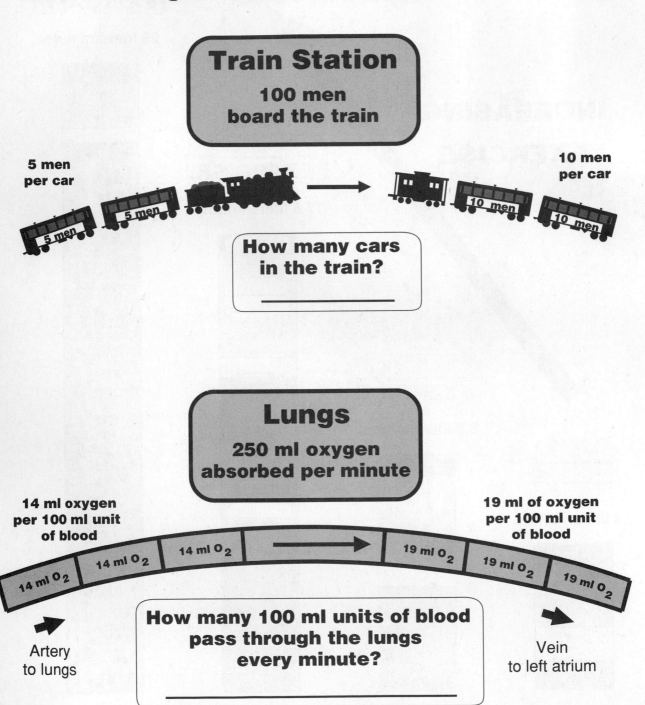

Train Station
100 men
board the train

5 men
per car

5 men

5 men

10 men
per car

10 men

10 men

**How many cars
in the train?**

_____

Lungs
250 ml oxygen
absorbed per minute

14 ml oxygen
per 100 ml unit
of blood

14 ml O_2

14 ml O_2

14 ml O_2

19 ml of oxygen
per 100 ml unit
of blood

19 ml O_2

19 ml O_2

19 ml O_2

Artery
to lungs

Vein
to left atrium

**How many 100 ml units of blood
pass through the lungs
every minute?**

_____

STROKE VOLUME (SV)

Relationship Between End–diastolic Volume and SV

At rest

> **Exercising**
> When more blood enters the ventricle, the ventricular muscle is stretched. It responds with a _____.

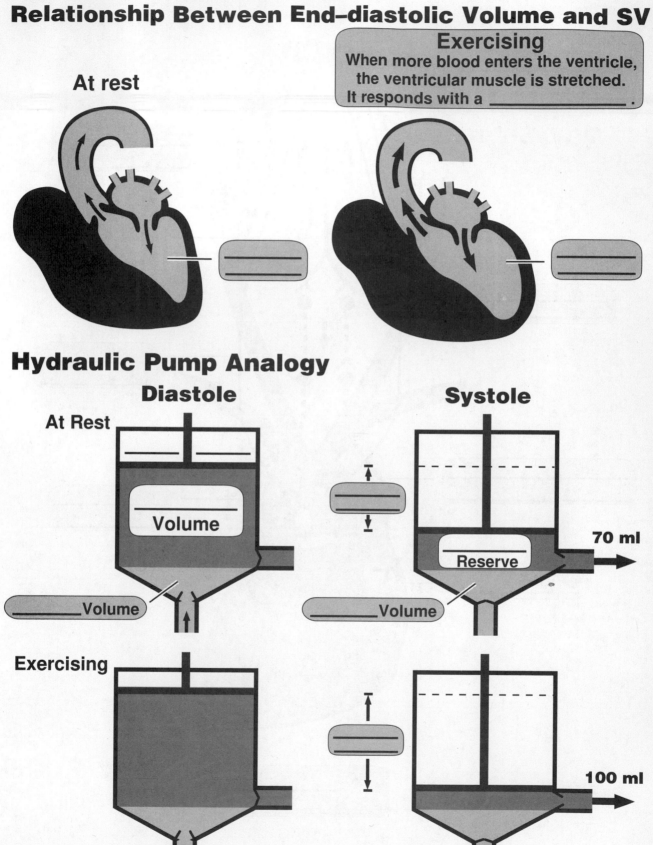

Hydraulic Pump Analogy

Diastole

At Rest

Volume

_____ Volume

Systole

70 ml

Reserve

_____ Volume

Exercising

100 ml

HEART RATE: Sympathetic Control

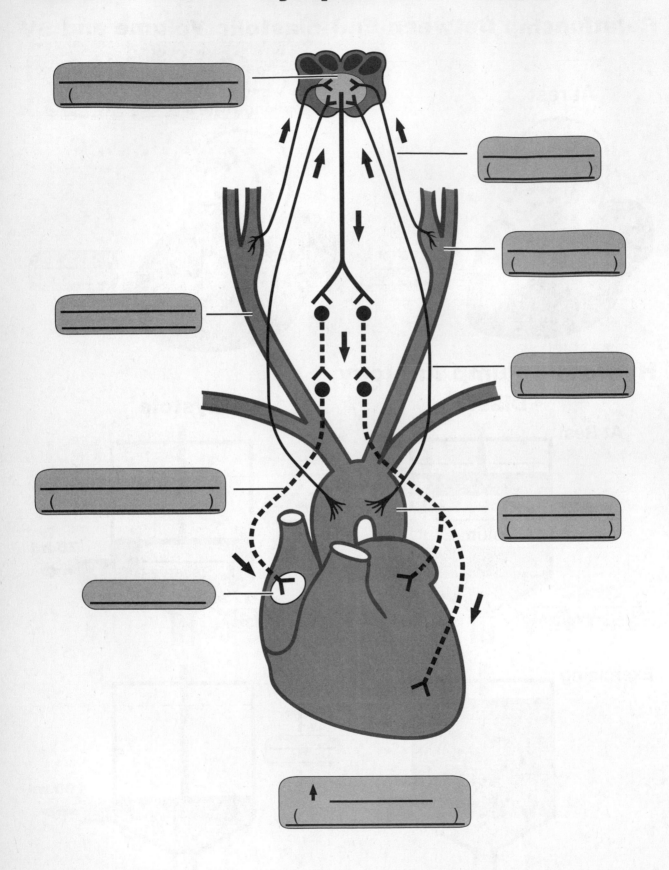

BLOOD VESSEL WALLS

**All blood vessel walls (except capillaries)
are composed of three basic tissue layers**

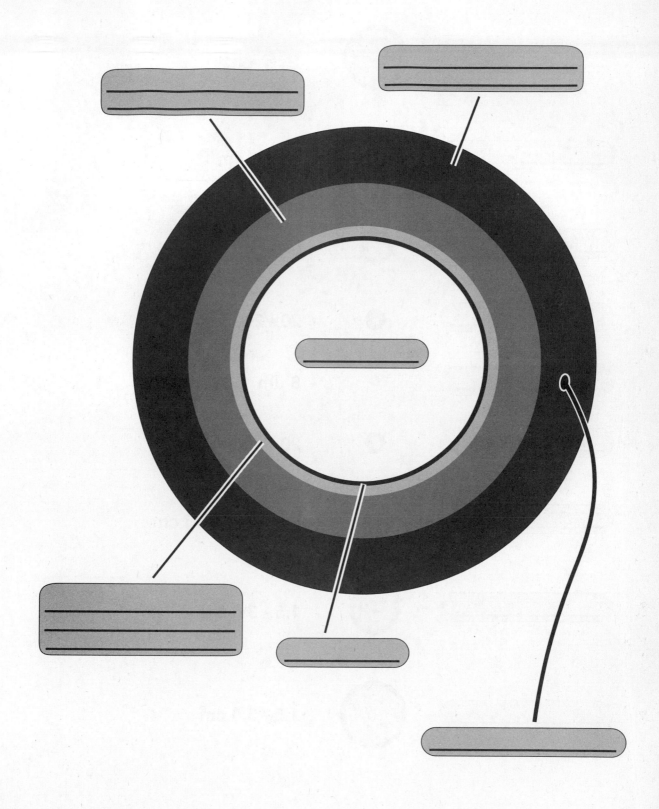

BLOOD VESSEL DIAMETERS
Lumen Diameters

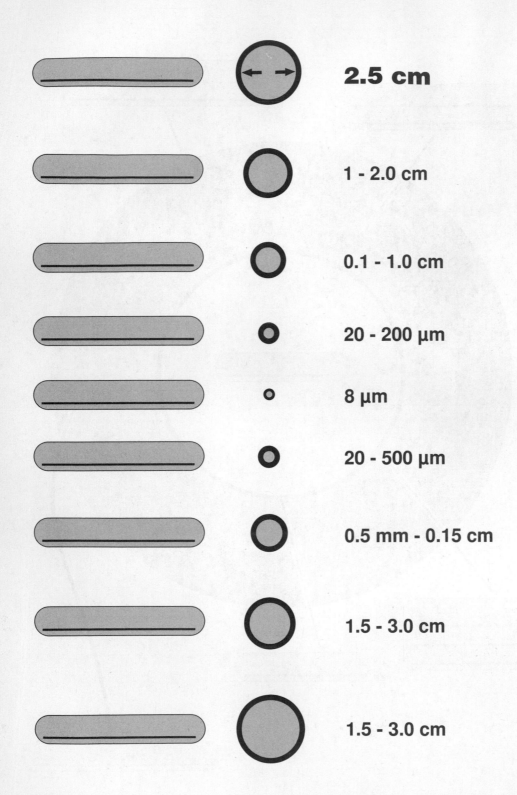

2.5 cm

1 - 2.0 cm

0.1 - 1.0 cm

20 - 200 µm

8 µm

20 - 500 µm

0.5 mm - 0.15 cm

1.5 - 3.0 cm

1.5 - 3.0 cm

BLOOD VESSEL WALL COMPOSITION

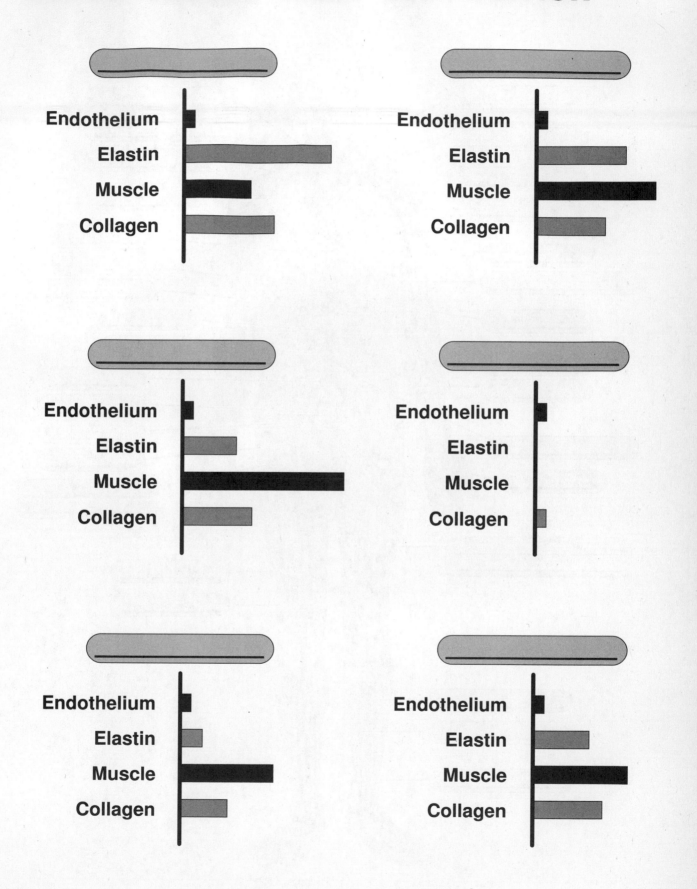

MAJOR ARTERIES

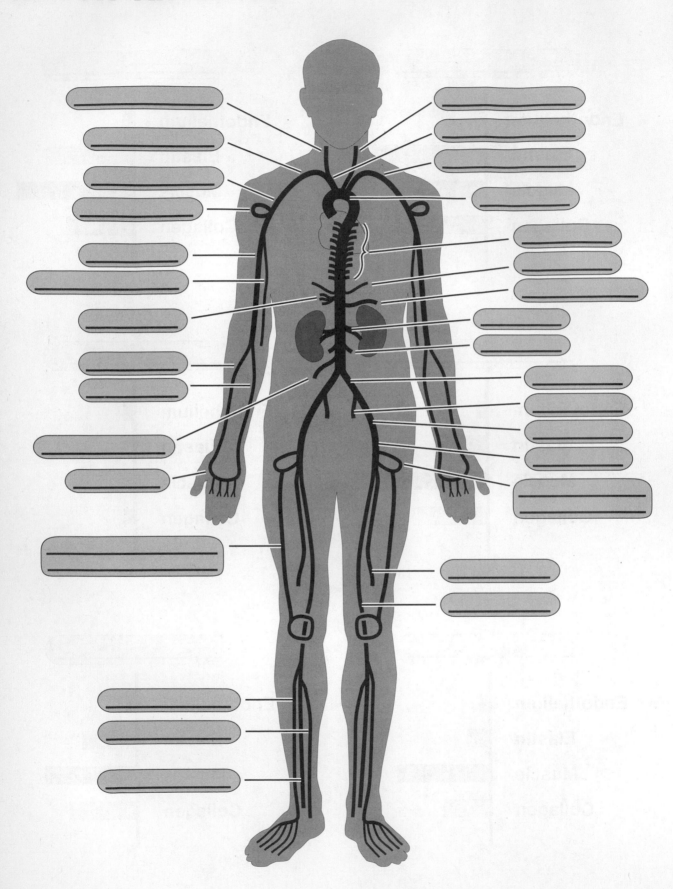

ELASTIC ARTERIES : elastic recoil
Schematic Illustration of Atrium, Ventricle, and Elastic Arteries

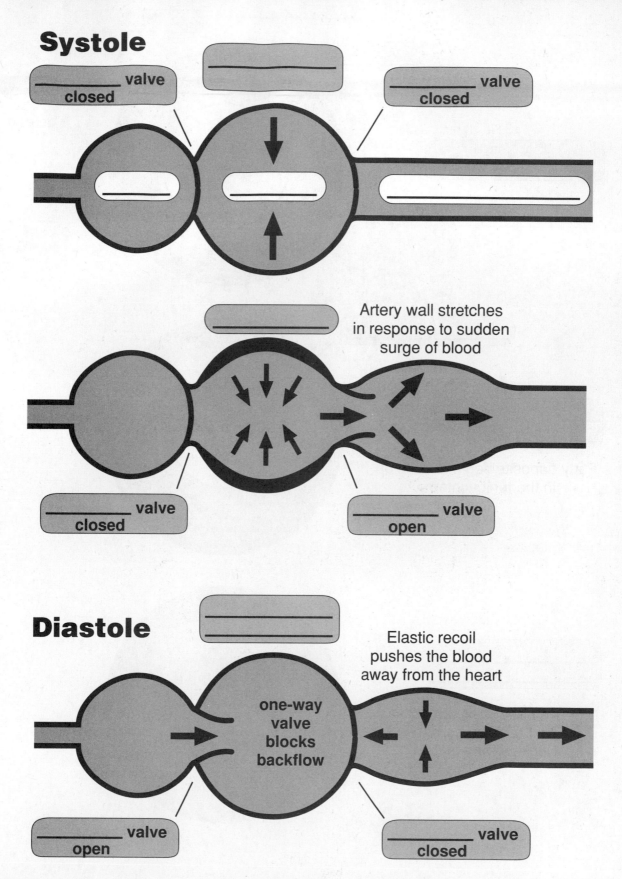

Systole

_____ valve
closed

_____ valve
closed

Artery wall stretches
in response to sudden
surge of blood

_____ valve
closed

_____ valve
open

Diastole

Elastic recoil
pushes the blood
away from the heart

one-way
valve
blocks
backflow

_____ valve
open

_____ valve
closed

135

ATHEROSCLEROSIS

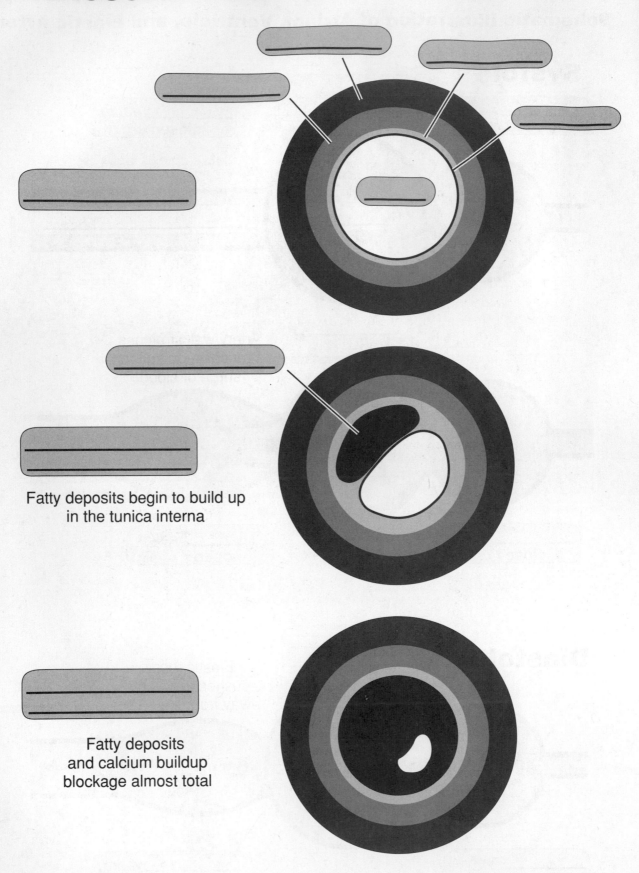

Fatty deposits begin to build up
in the tunica interna

Fatty deposits
and calcium buildup
blockage almost total

ARTERIOLE

The lumen diameter of arterioles regulates the _____ of blood and helps maintain the normal _____ .

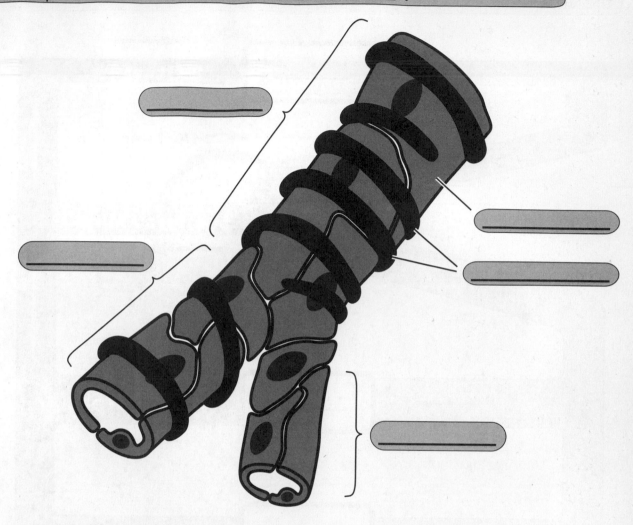

Lumen Diameter

The lumen diameter is inversely proportional to the frequency of _____ nerve impulses.

Diameter Range : 20 - 200 μm

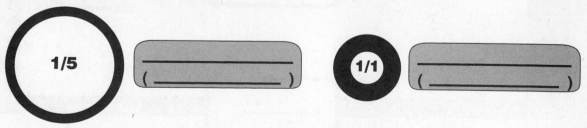

1/5

1/1

ARTERIOLES : Distribution of Blood

The lumen diameters of the _____ leading to an organ determine the volume of blood flow to that organ.

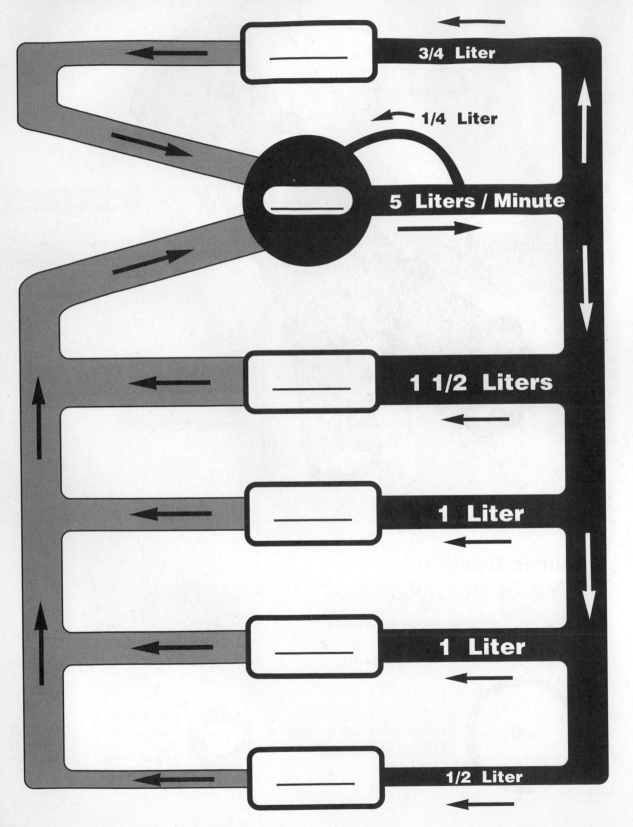

3/4 Liter

1/4 Liter

5 Liters / Minute

1 1/2 Liters

1 Liter

1 Liter

1/2 Liter

ARTERIOLES : Distribution of Blood to the Skin

Blood flow to the skin is regulated by the _____ diameters of the arterioles carrying blood to the skin.

The degree of _____ of the arterioles is directly proportional to the degree of stimulation by sympathetic nerves.

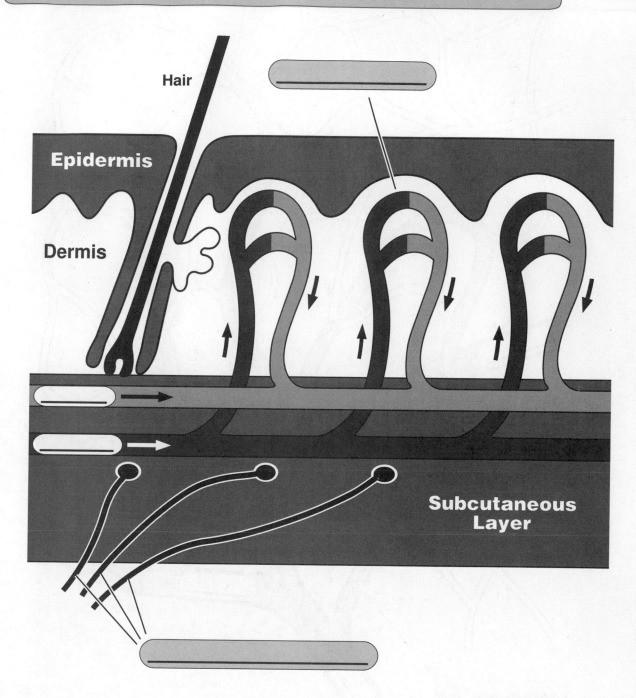

Hair

Epidermis

Dermis

Subcutaneous Layer

CAPILLARY BED

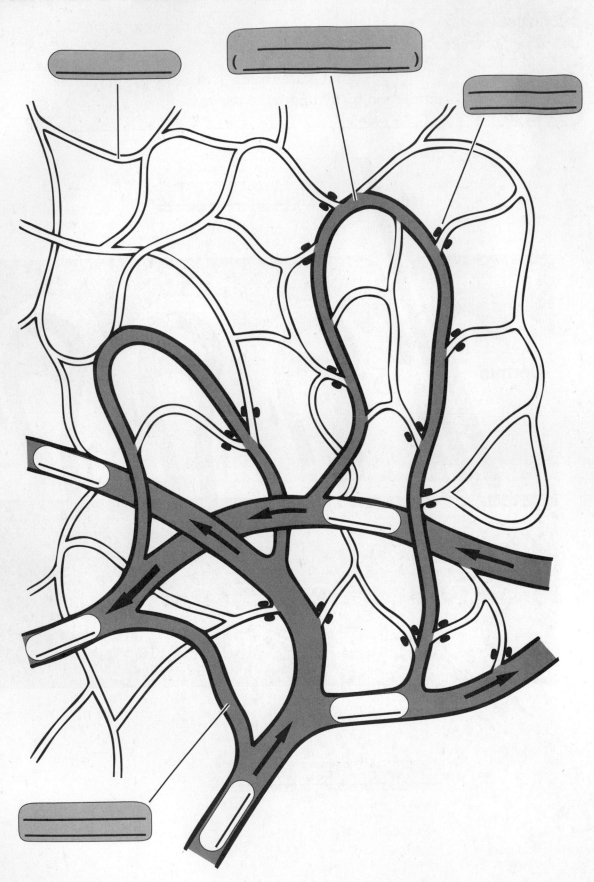

CAPILLARY
Cross Section

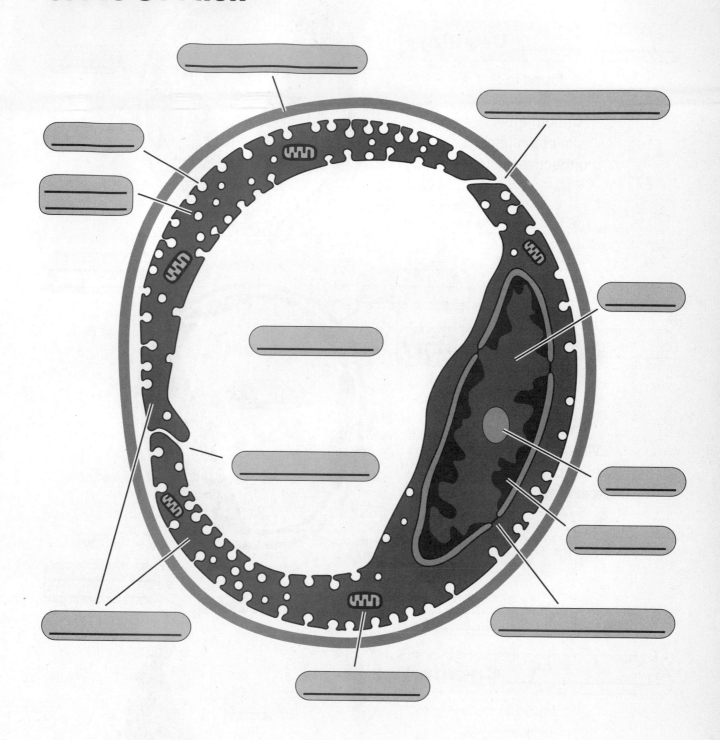

TYPES OF CAPILLARIES

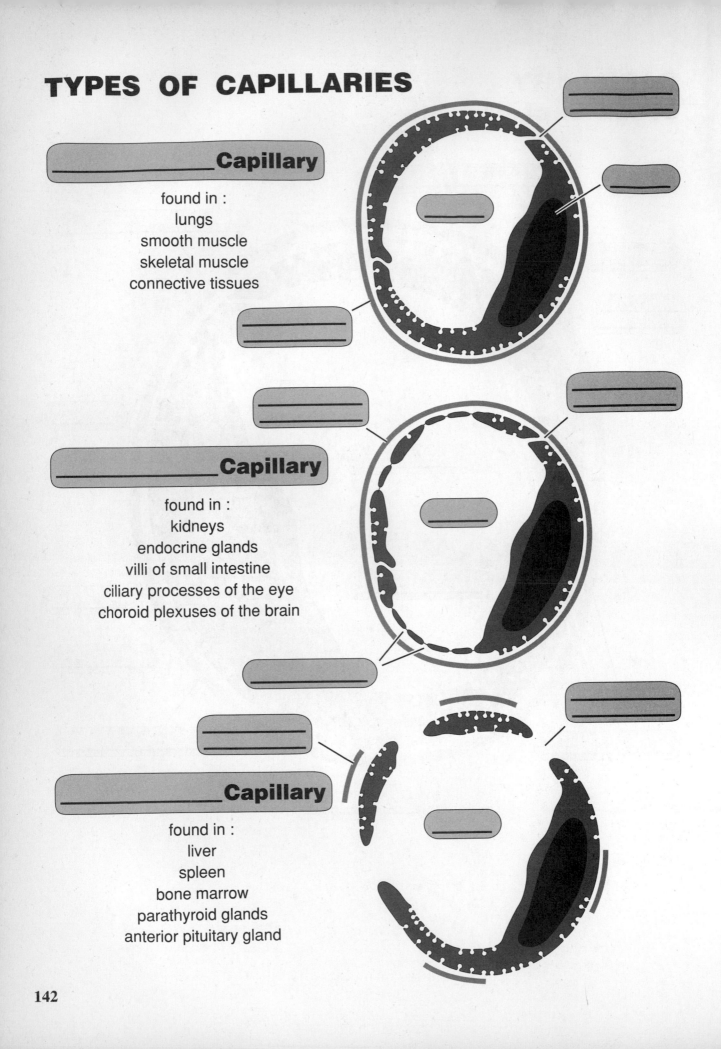

_____ Capillary

found in :
lungs
smooth muscle
skeletal muscle
connective tissues

_____ Capillary

found in :
kidneys
endocrine glands
villi of small intestine
ciliary processes of the eye
choroid plexuses of the brain

_____ Capillary

found in :
liver
spleen
bone marrow
parathyroid glands
anterior pituitary gland

CAPILLARY : Exchange of Food and Waste

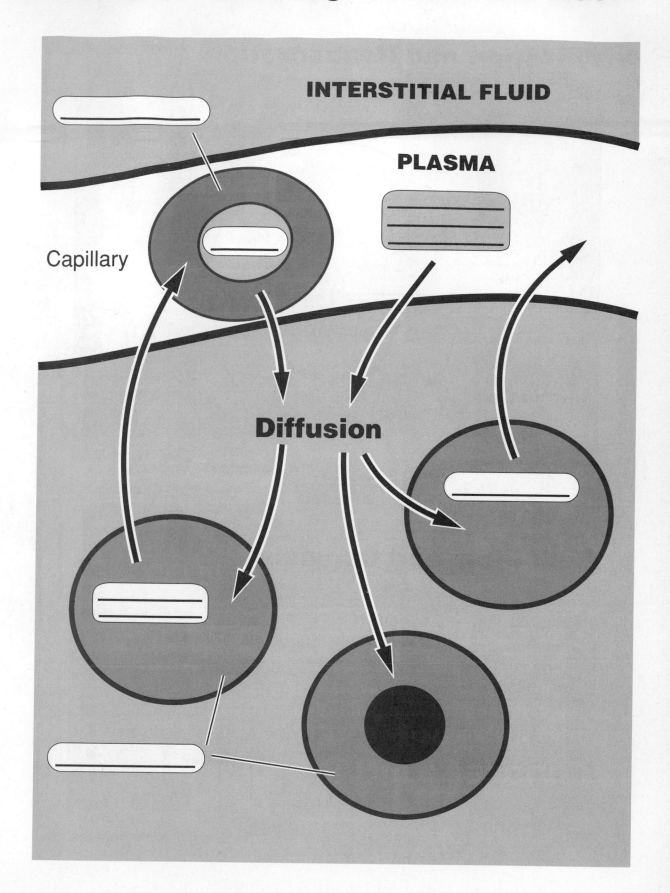

INTERSTITIAL FLUID

PLASMA

Capillary

Diffusion

CAPILLARY : Exchange of Fluid

Filtration and Reabsorption

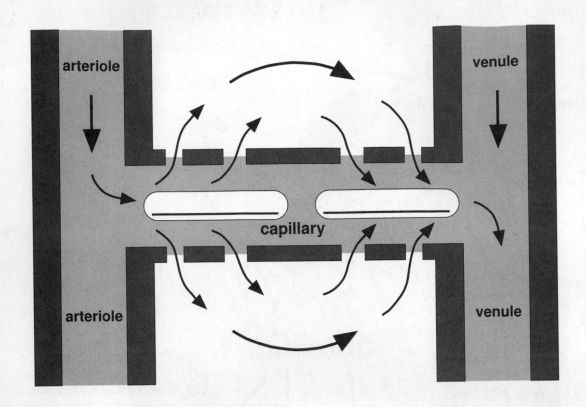

Bulk Flow and Osmosis

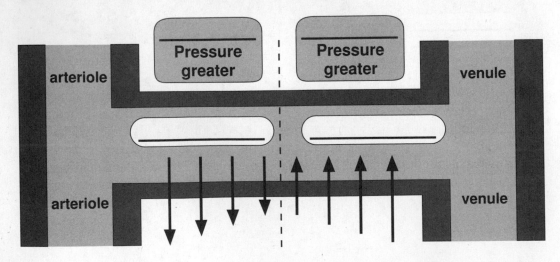

CAPILLARY: PRESSURE GRADIENTS

Numbers : the pressure in mm Hg.
Arrows : the direction that fluid moves.

BHP : _____
IFOP : _____
BCOP : _____

Hydrostatic Pressures

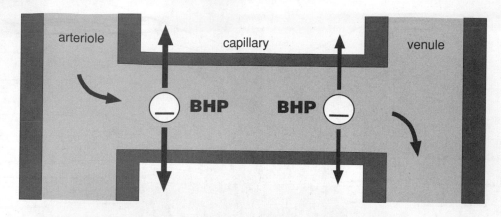

Osmotic Pressures (average values)

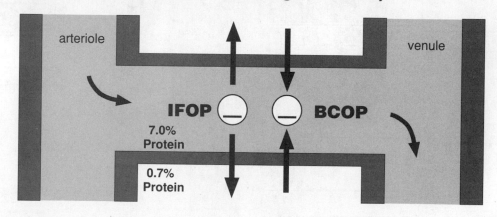

Net Pressures = _____ **+** _____ **−** _____

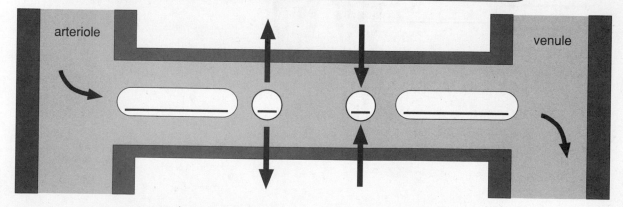

MAJOR VEINS

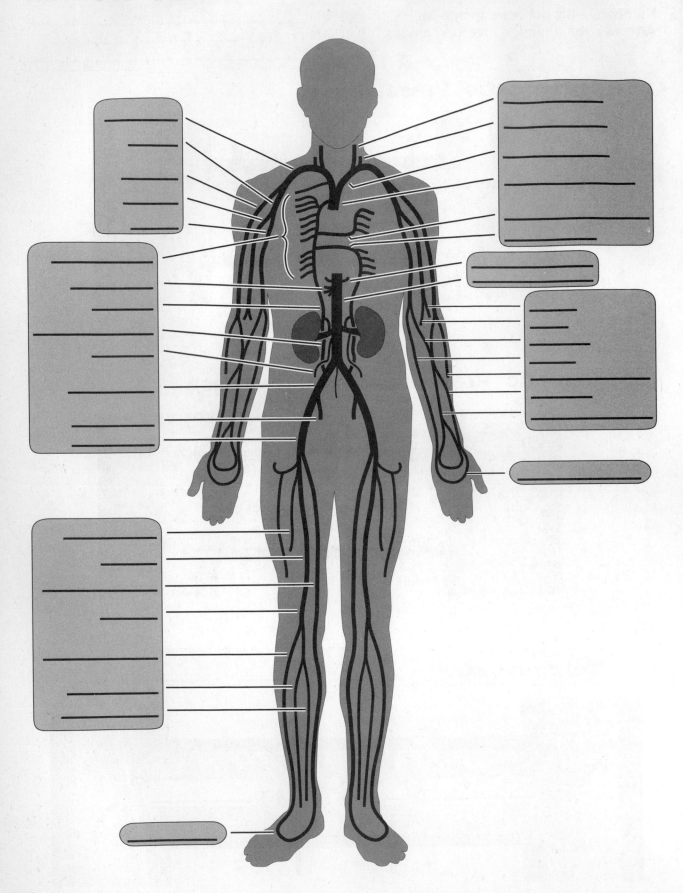

VENOUS RETURN
Body Cavities

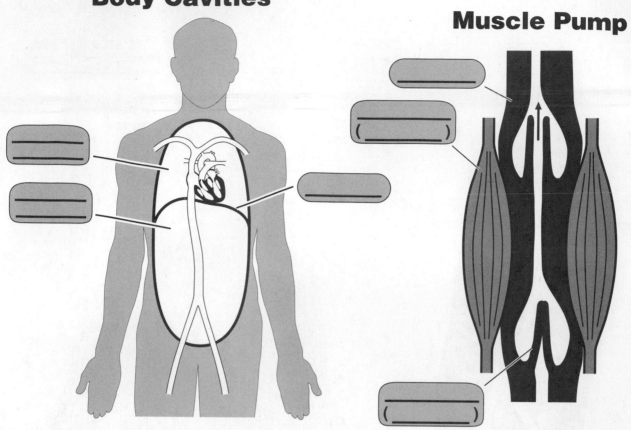

Muscle Pump

Respiratory Pump

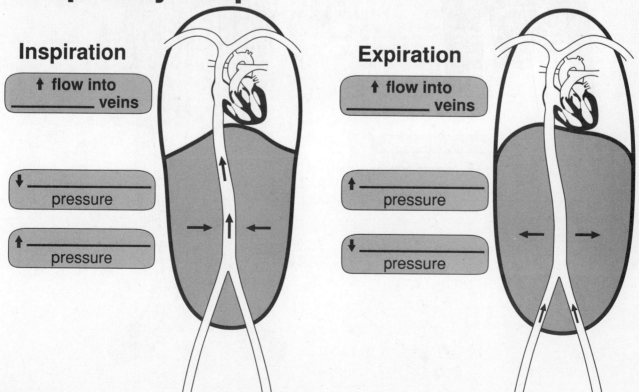

Inspiration

↑ flow into
_____ veins

↓ _____
pressure

↑ _____
pressure

Expiration

↑ flow into
_____ veins

↑ _____
pressure

↓ _____
pressure

LYMPHATIC VESSELS

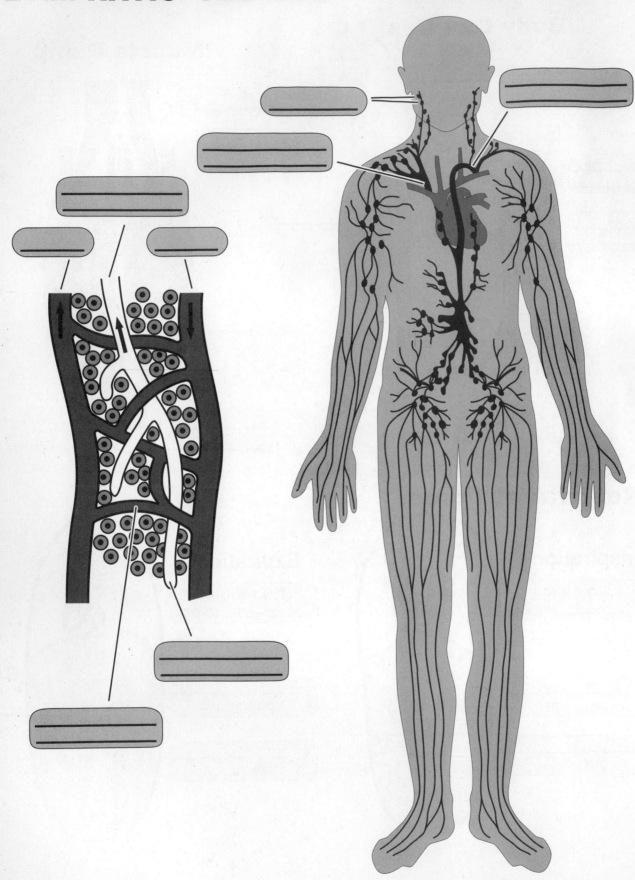

ARTERIES : Heart

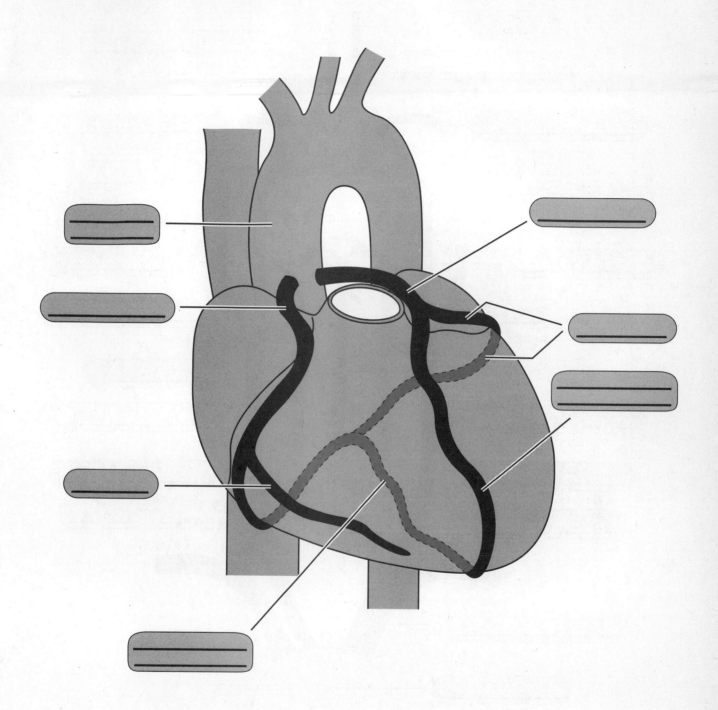

ARTERIES : Brain

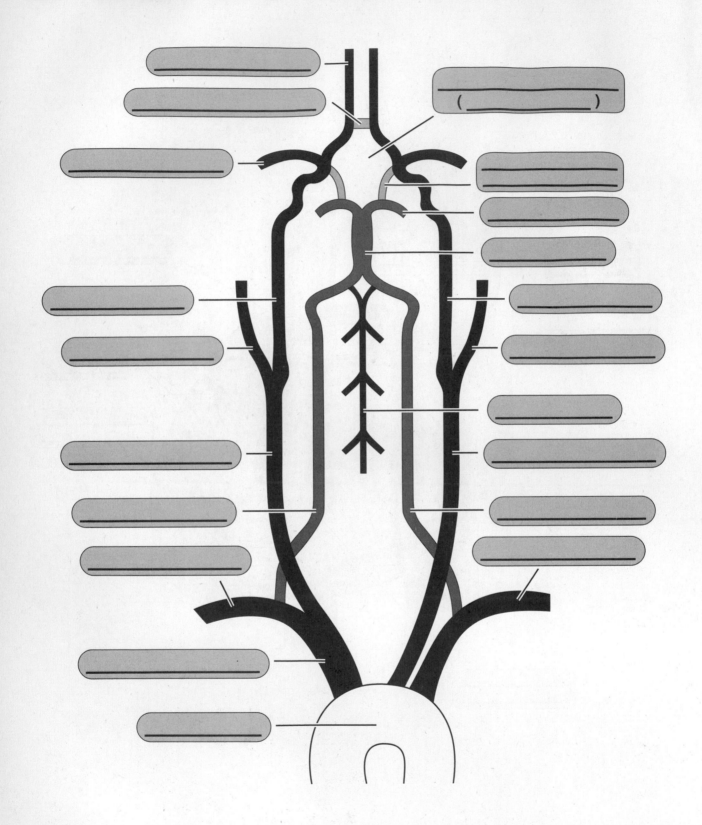

ARTERIES : Right Upper Extremity

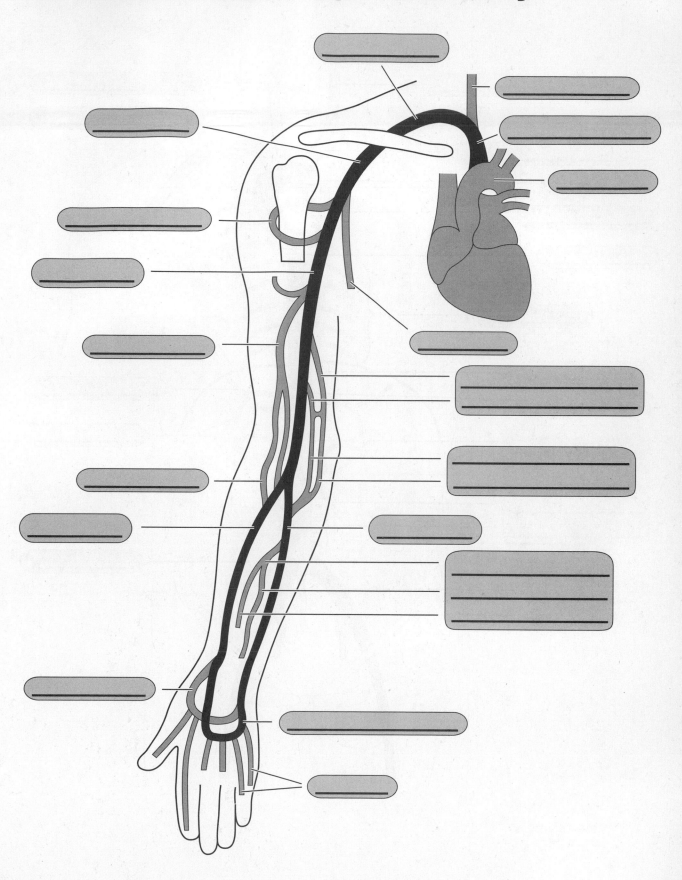

ARTERIES : Aorta and Its Major Branches

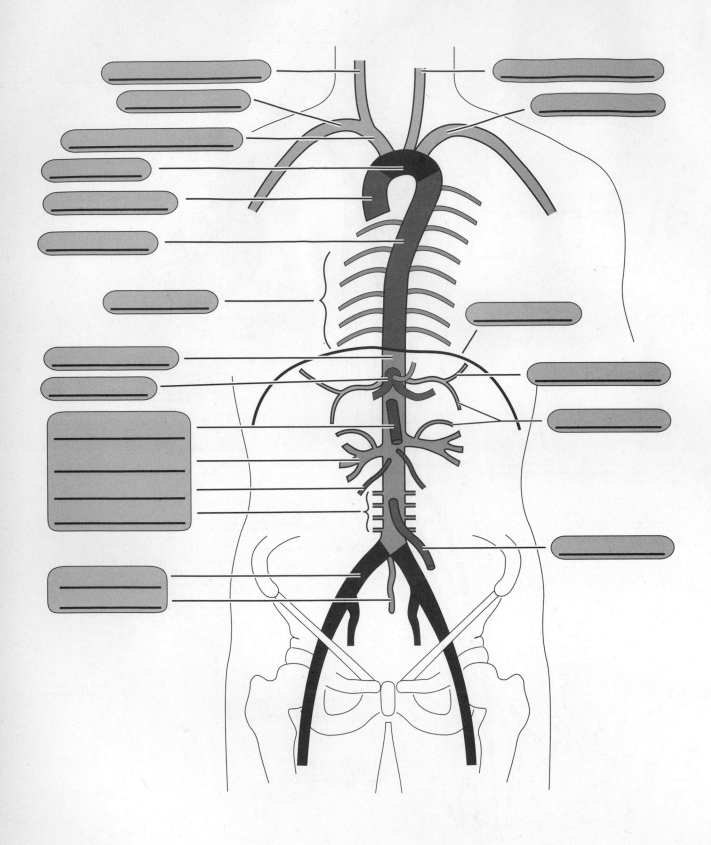

ARTERIES : Celiac Trunk

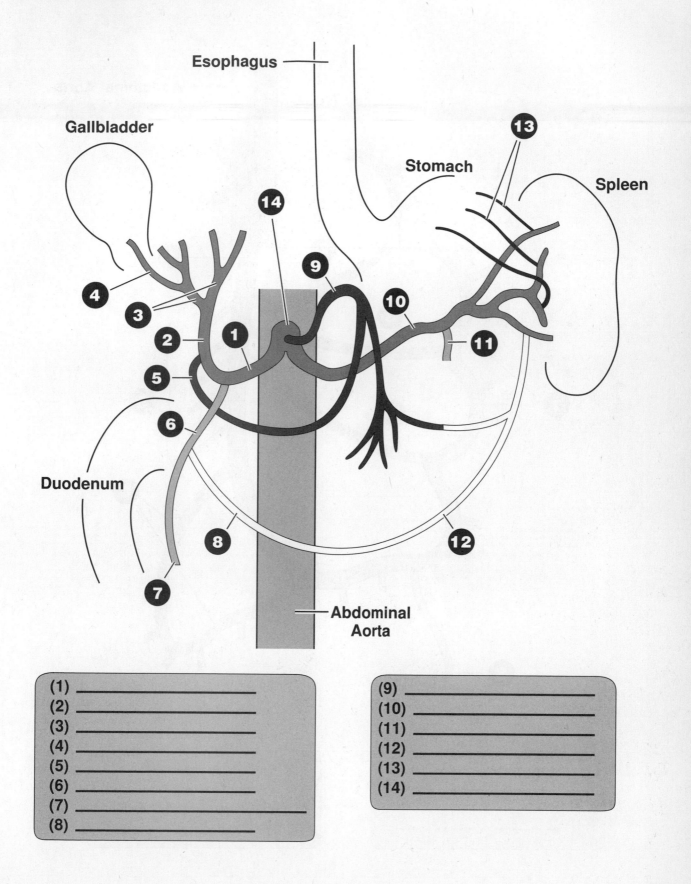

Esophagus

Gallbladder

Stomach

Spleen

⑬

⑭

⑨

④

⑩

③

②

①

⑤

⑪

⑥

Duodenum

⑧

⑫

⑦

Abdominal
Aorta

(1) _____
(2) _____
(3) _____
(4) _____
(5) _____
(6) _____
(7) _____
(8) _____

(9) _____
(10) _____
(11) _____
(12) _____
(13) _____
(14) _____

ARTERIES : Superior Mesenteric

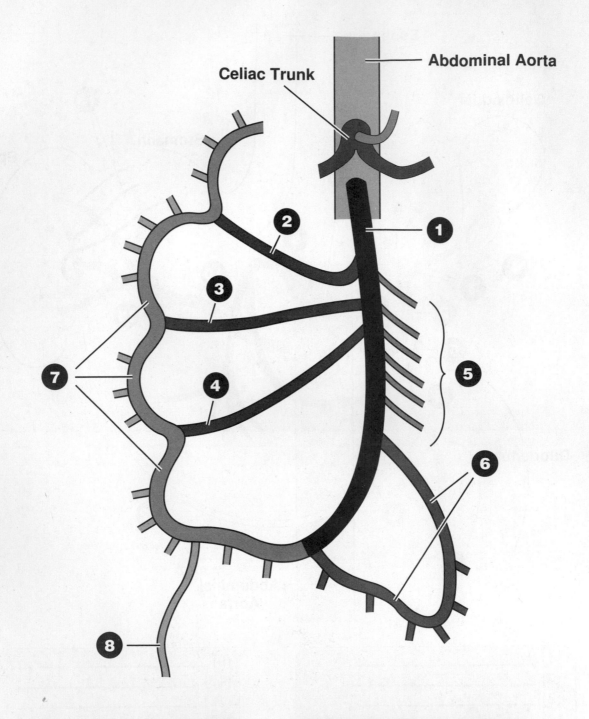

Celiac Trunk

Abdominal Aorta

(1) _____
(2) _____
(3) _____
(4) _____

(5) _____
(6) _____
(7) _____
(8) _____

ARTERIES : Inferior Mesenteric

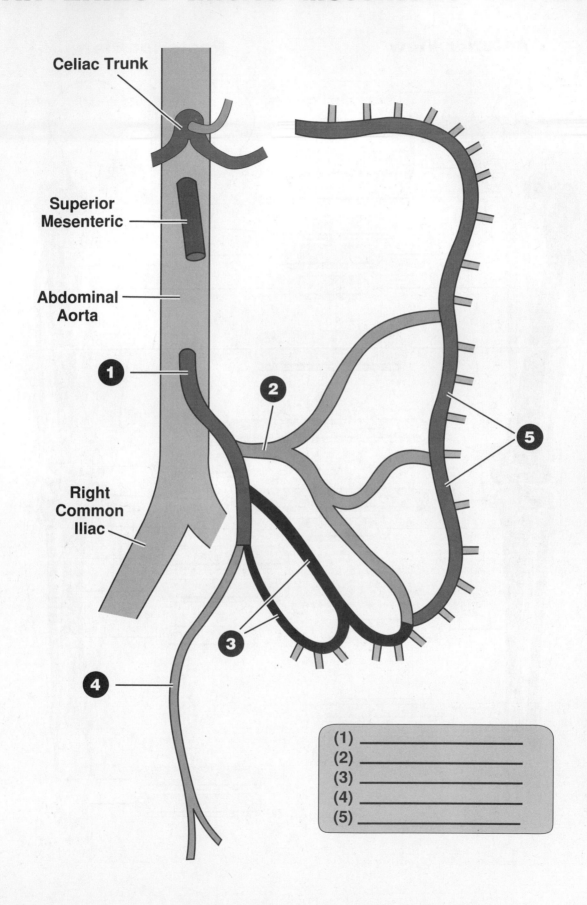

Celiac Trunk

Superior
Mesenteric

Abdominal
Aorta

Right
Common
Iliac

(1) _____
(2) _____
(3) _____
(4) _____
(5) _____

ARTERIES : Lower Extremity

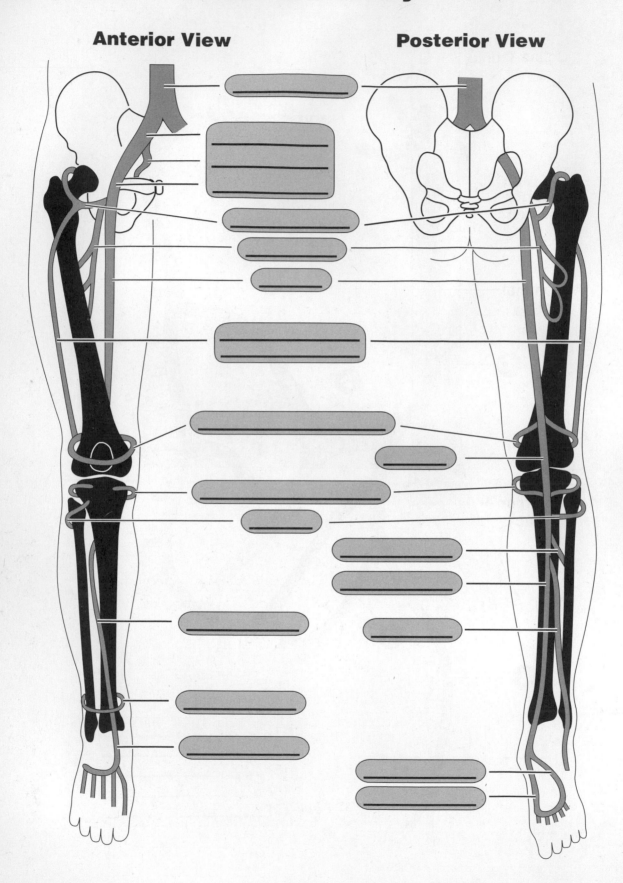

156

VEINS : Heart

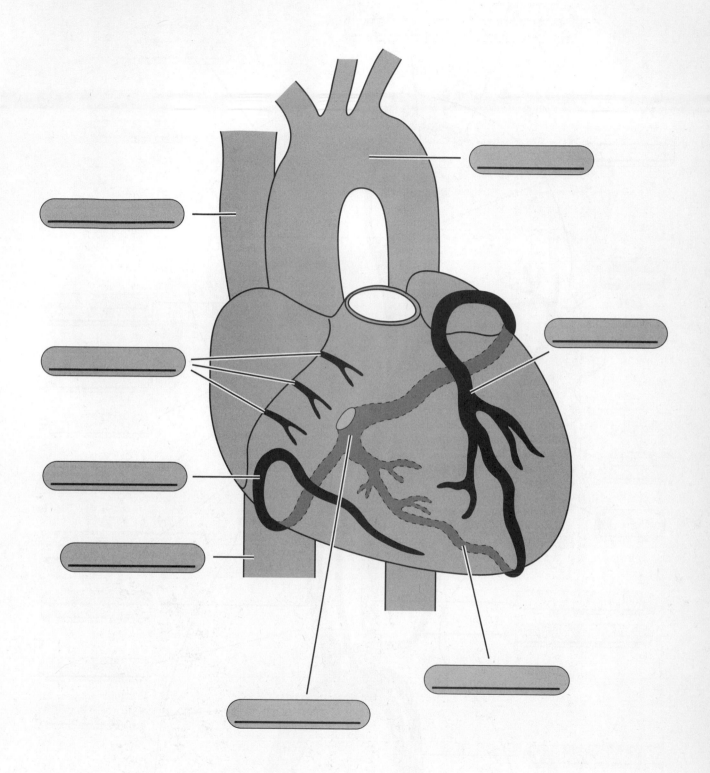

VEINS : Brain

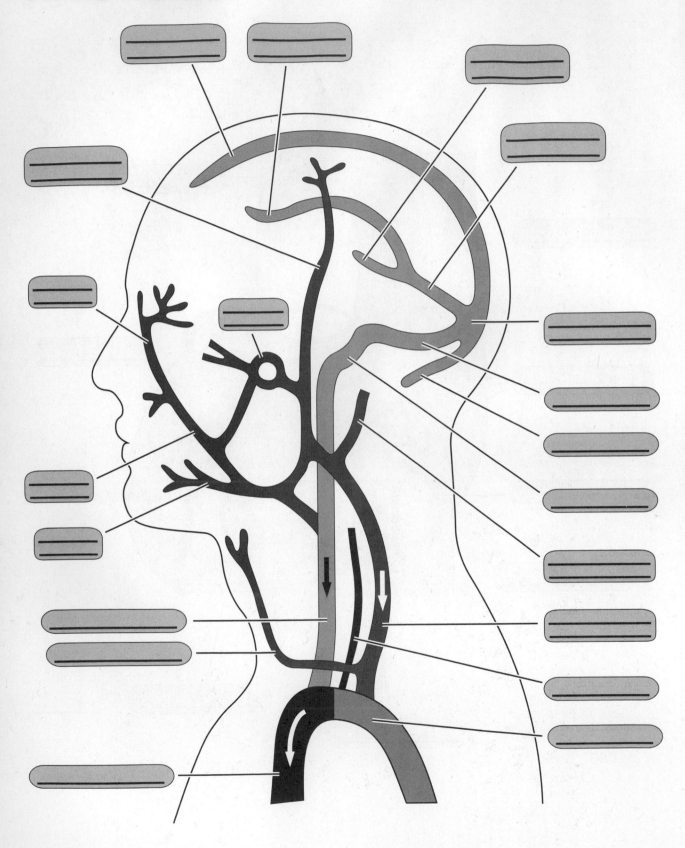

VEINS : Upper Extremity

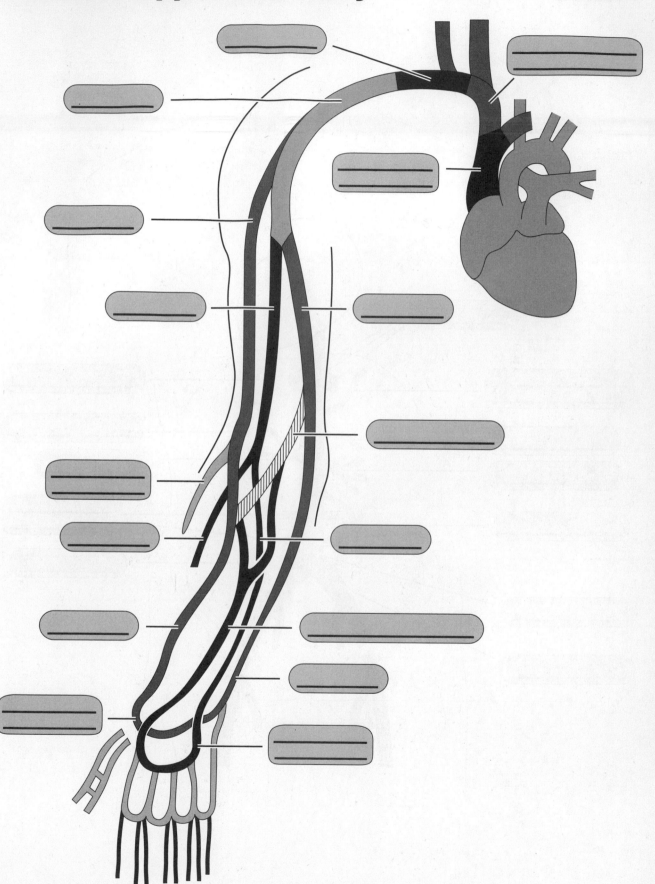

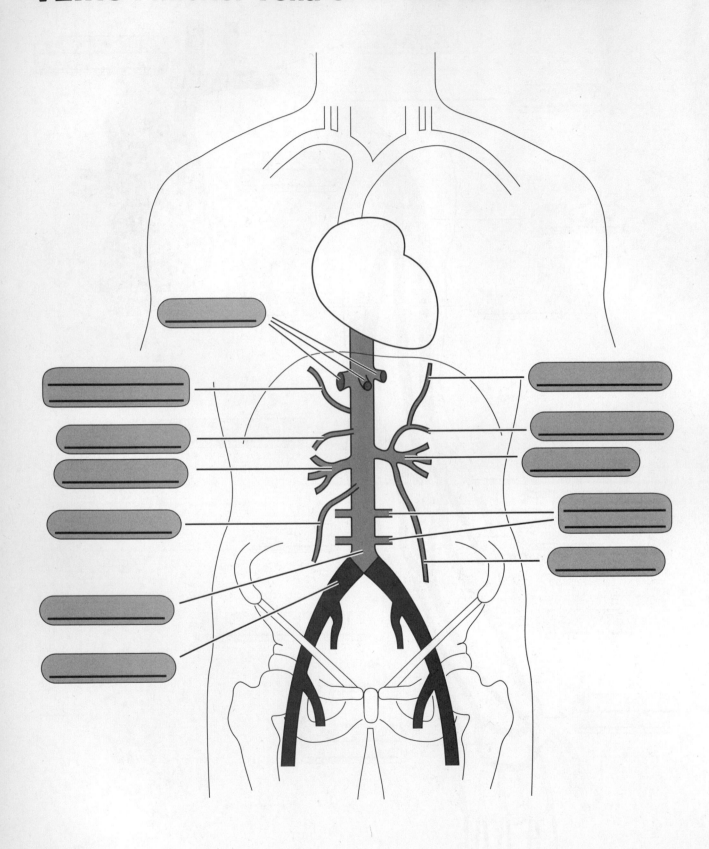

VEINS : Azygos System

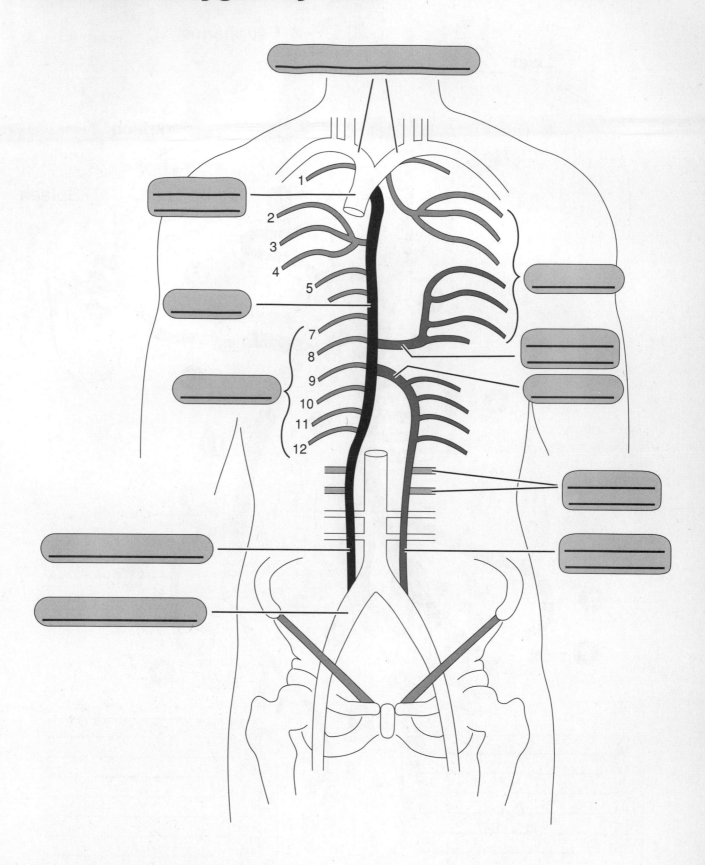

1
2
3
4
5
7
8
9
10
11
12

VEINS : Hepatic Portal System

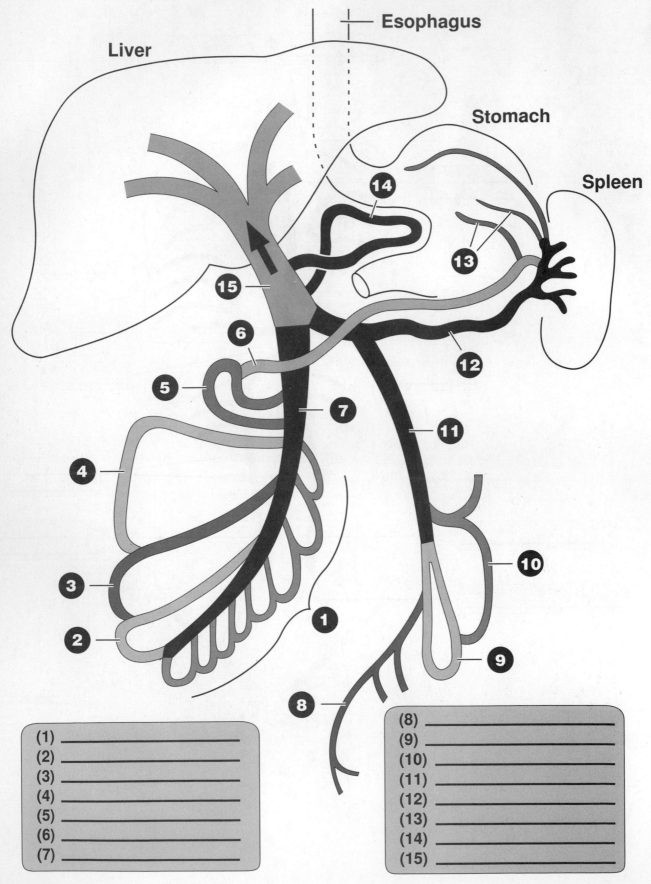

Esophagus

Liver

Stomach

Spleen

(1) _____
(2) _____
(3) _____
(4) _____
(5) _____
(6) _____
(7) _____

(8) _____
(9) _____
(10) _____
(11) _____
(12) _____
(13) _____
(14) _____
(15) _____

VEINS : Lower Extremity

Anterior View

Posterior View

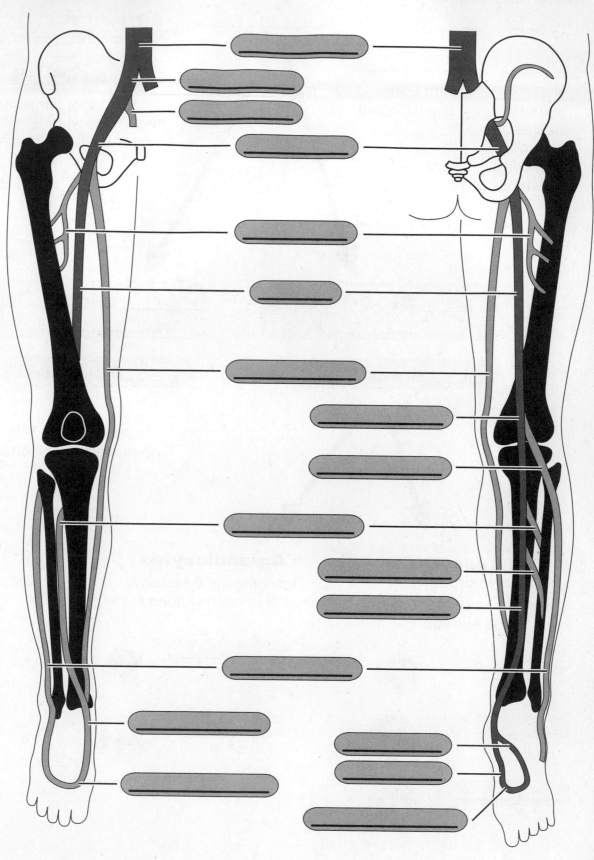

BLOOD COMPOSITION

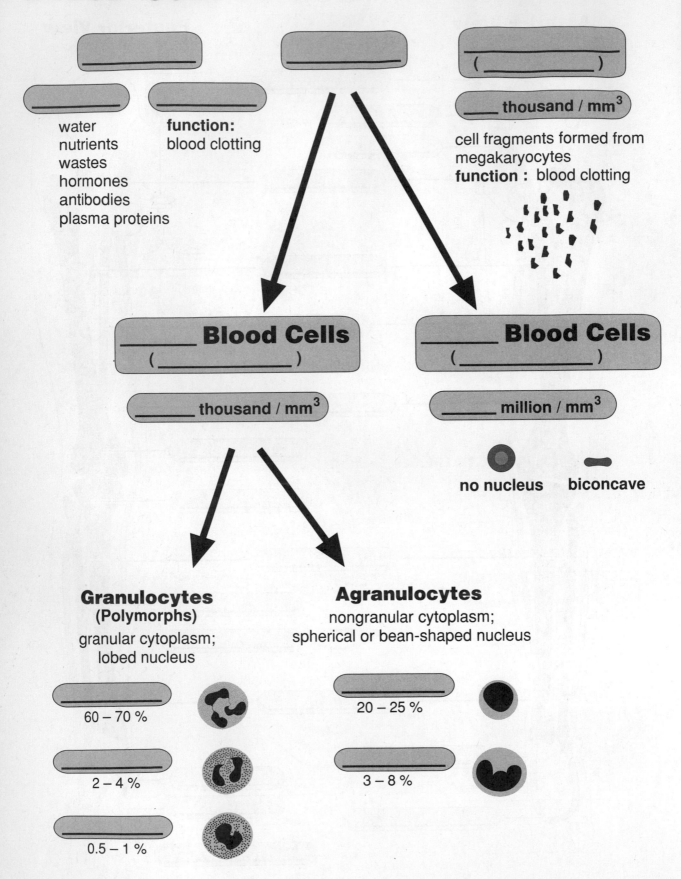

_____

_____

_____

_____

(_____)

_____ thousand / mm³

water
nutrients
wastes
hormones
antibodies
plasma proteins

function:
blood clotting

cell fragments formed from
megakaryocytes
function : blood clotting

_____ **Blood Cells**
(_____)

_____ **Blood Cells**
(_____)

_____ thousand / mm³

_____ million / mm³

no nucleus   biconcave

Granulocytes
(Polymorphs)

granular cytoplasm;
lobed nucleus

Agranulocytes

nongranular cytoplasm;
spherical or bean-shaped nucleus

_____
60 – 70 %

_____
20 – 25 %

_____
2 – 4 %

_____
3 – 8 %

_____
0.5 – 1 %

PLASMA

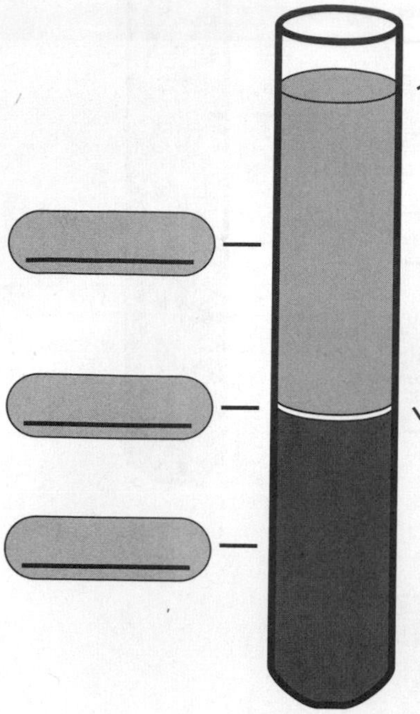

92 % of plasma

albumin
alpha globulins
beta globulins
gamma globulins
fibrinogen
prothrombin

nitrogen-containing compounds
carbohydrates
organic acids
lipids

salts : sodium, potassium, magnesium,
 & calcium chloride; sodium sulfate.
buffers : bicarbonate & phosphate buffers
gases : carbon dioxide, oxygen, & nitrogen

Electrolyte Composition of Blood Plasma

Cations (positively charged ions)

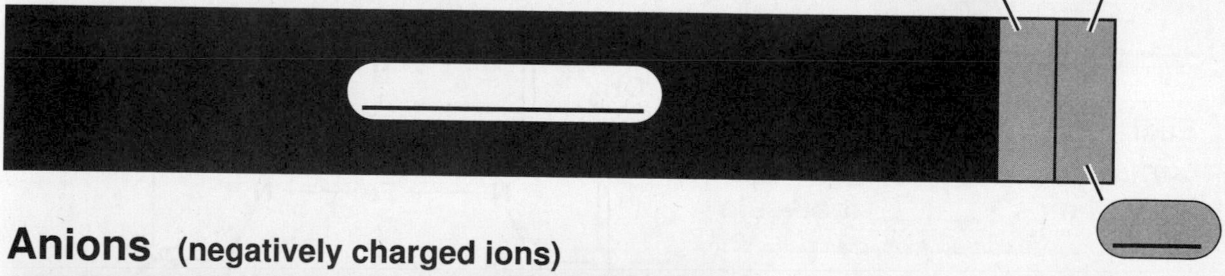

Anions (negatively charged ions)

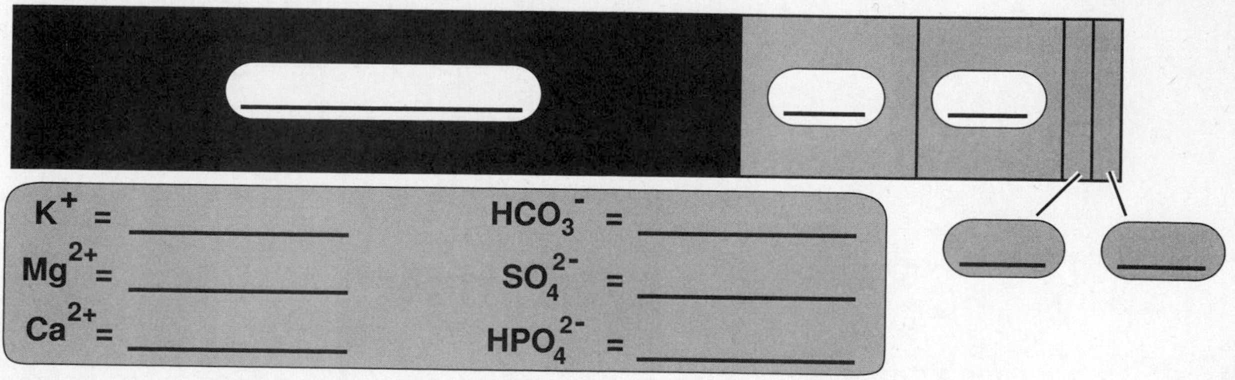

K^+ = _____

Mg^{2+} = _____

Ca^{2+} = _____

HCO_3^- = _____

SO_4^{2-} = _____

HPO_4^{2-} = _____

RED BLOOD CELLS

(_____)

(schematic)

Hematocrit
Percent of RBCs
by Volume

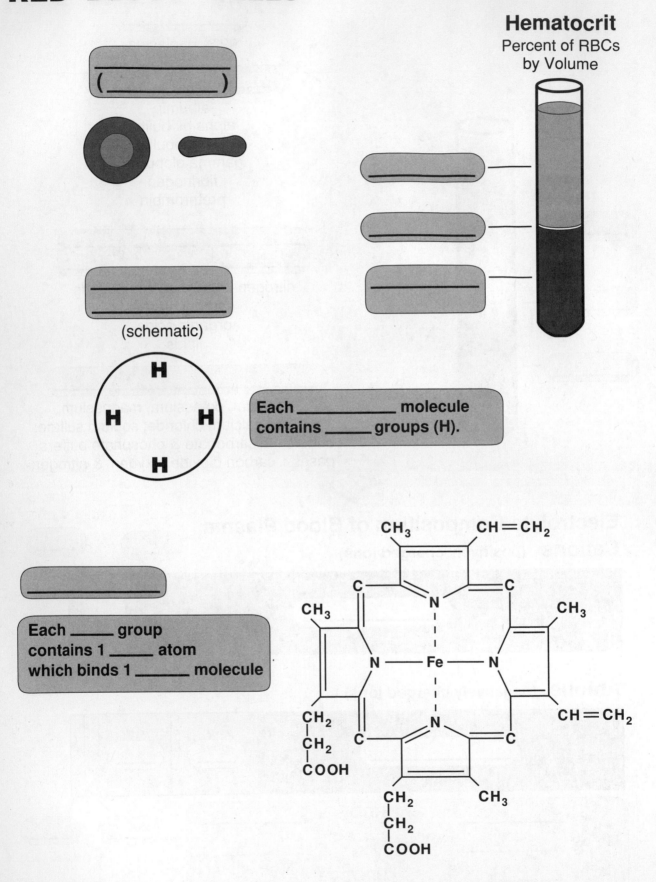

Each _____ molecule
contains _____ groups (H).

Each _____ group
contains 1 _____ atom
which binds 1 _____ molecule

WHITE BLOOD CELLS

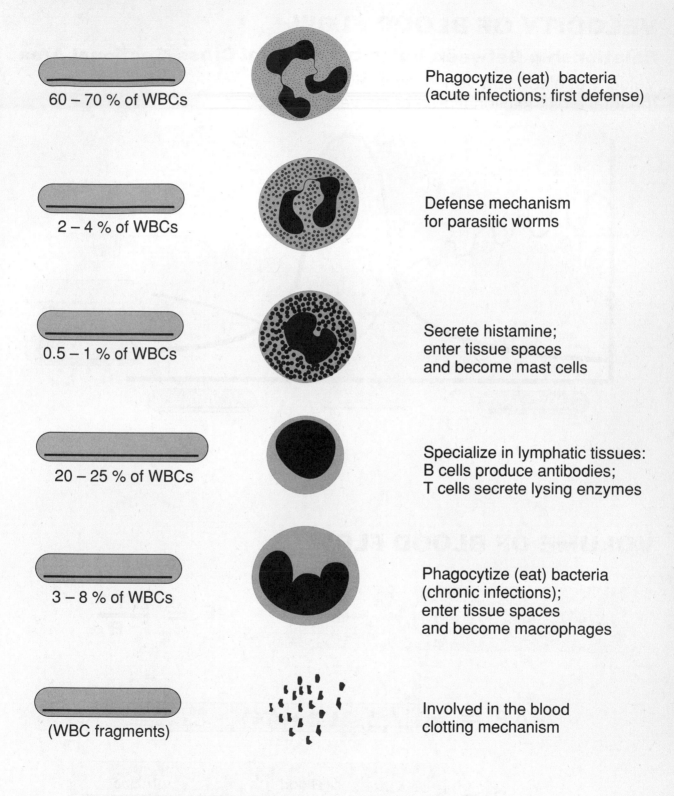

60 – 70 % of WBCs

Phagocytize (eat) bacteria
(acute infections; first defense)

2 – 4 % of WBCs

Defense mechanism
for parasitic worms

0.5 – 1 % of WBCs

Secrete histamine;
enter tissue spaces
and become mast cells

20 – 25 % of WBCs

Specialize in lymphatic tissues:
B cells produce antibodies;
T cells secrete lysing enzymes

3 – 8 % of WBCs

Phagocytize (eat) bacteria
(chronic infections);
enter tissue spaces
and become macrophages

(WBC fragments)

Involved in the blood
clotting mechanism

HEMODYNAMICS

VELOCITY OF BLOOD FLOW
Relationship Between Velocity and Total Cross–Sectional Area

Velocity of blood flow varies inversely with
the total cross-sectional area of the vessels.

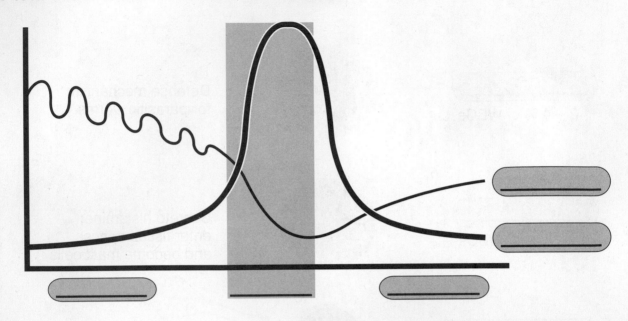

VOLUME OF BLOOD FLOW

$$\text{Flow} = \underline{\hspace{4cm}} \qquad F = \frac{\Delta P}{R}$$

$$\Delta P = \underline{\hspace{3cm}} \text{ Pressure} - \underline{\hspace{2.5cm}} \text{ Pressure}$$

$$R = \frac{\underline{\hspace{2cm}} \text{ of Blood } \times \underline{\hspace{1.5cm}} \text{ of Tube}}{(\underline{\hspace{2cm}} \text{ of Lumen})^4}$$

PRESSURE CHANGES IN THE SYSTEMIC CIRCULATION

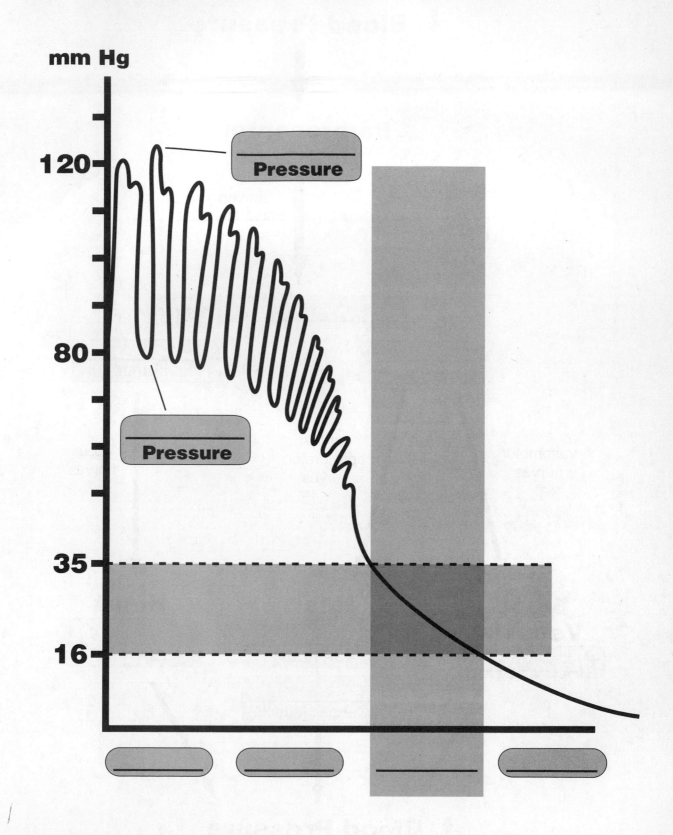

BLOOD PRESSURE : Neural Regulation

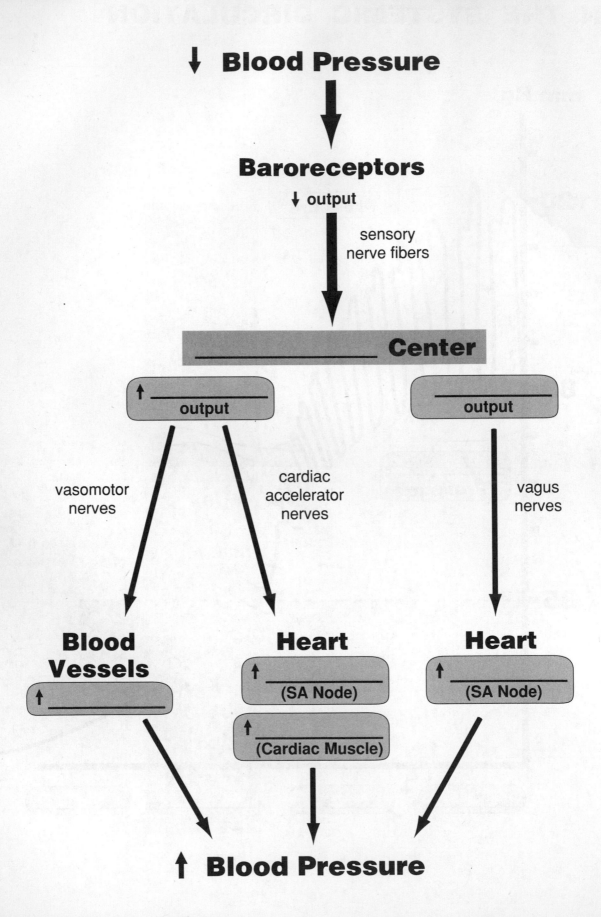

↓ **Blood Pressure**

Baroreceptors

↓ output

sensory
nerve fibers

_____ **Center**

↑ _____ output

_____ output

vasomotor
nerves

cardiac
accelerator
nerves

vagus
nerves

**Blood
Vessels**

↑ _____

Heart

↑ _____
(SA Node)

↑ _____
(Cardiac Muscle)

Heart

↑ _____
(SA Node)

↑ **Blood Pressure**

BLOOD PRESSURE : Hormonal Regulation

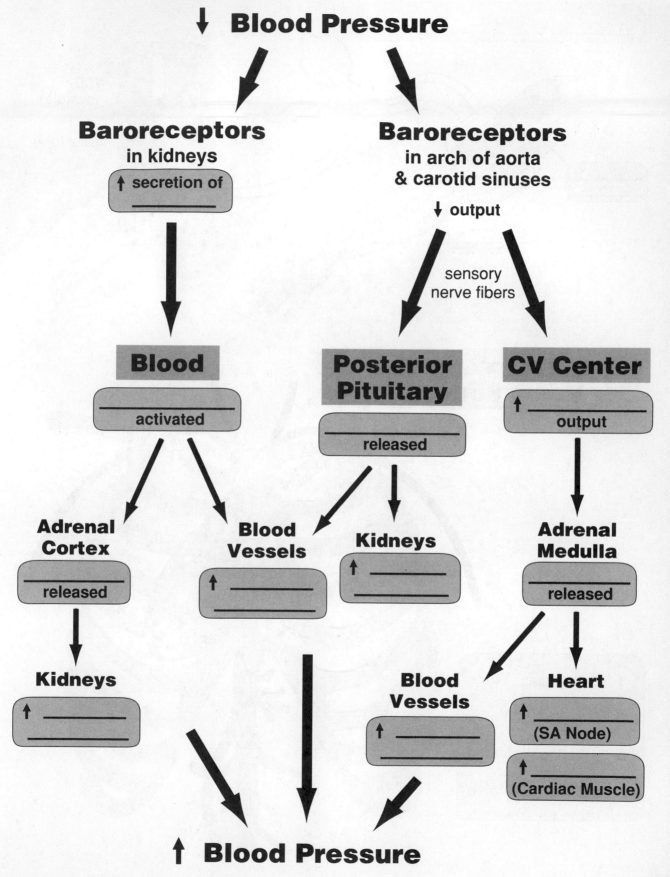

↓ **Blood Pressure**

Baroreceptors
in kidneys

↑ secretion of
_____

Baroreceptors
in arch of aorta
& carotid sinuses

↓ output

sensory
nerve fibers

Blood

_____
activated

**Posterior
Pituitary**

_____
released

CV Center

↑ _____
output

**Adrenal
Cortex**

_____
released

**Blood
Vessels**

↑ _____

Kidneys

↑ _____
_____

**Adrenal
Medulla**

_____
released

Kidneys

↑ _____
_____

**Blood
Vessels**

↑ _____
_____

Heart

↑ _____
(SA Node)

↑ _____
(Cardiac Muscle)

↑ **Blood Pressure**

MEASUREMENT OF BLOOD PRESSURE

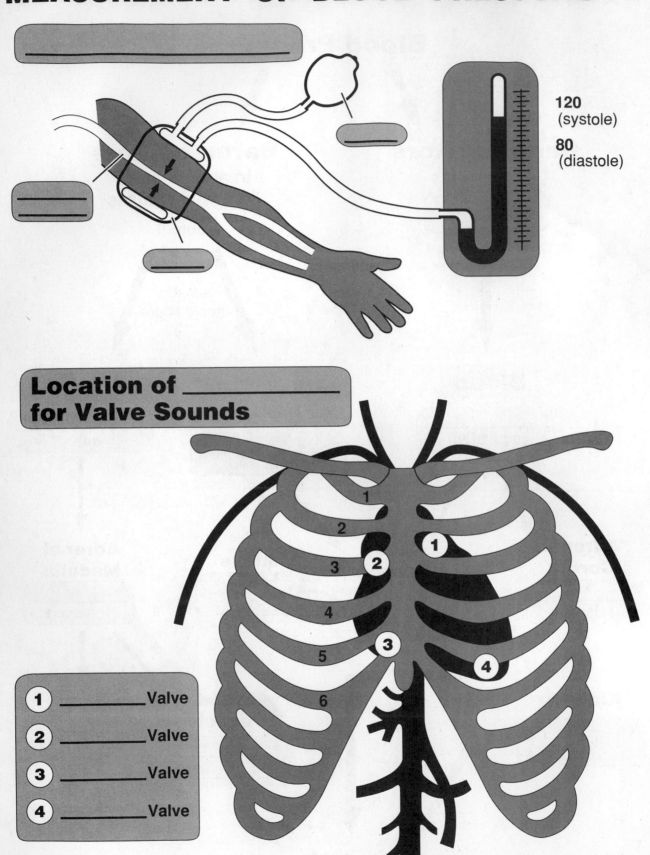

120 (systole)

80 (diastole)

Location of _____ for Valve Sounds

1 _____ Valve
2 _____ Valve
3 _____ Valve
4 _____ Valve

BLOOD CLOT FORMATION

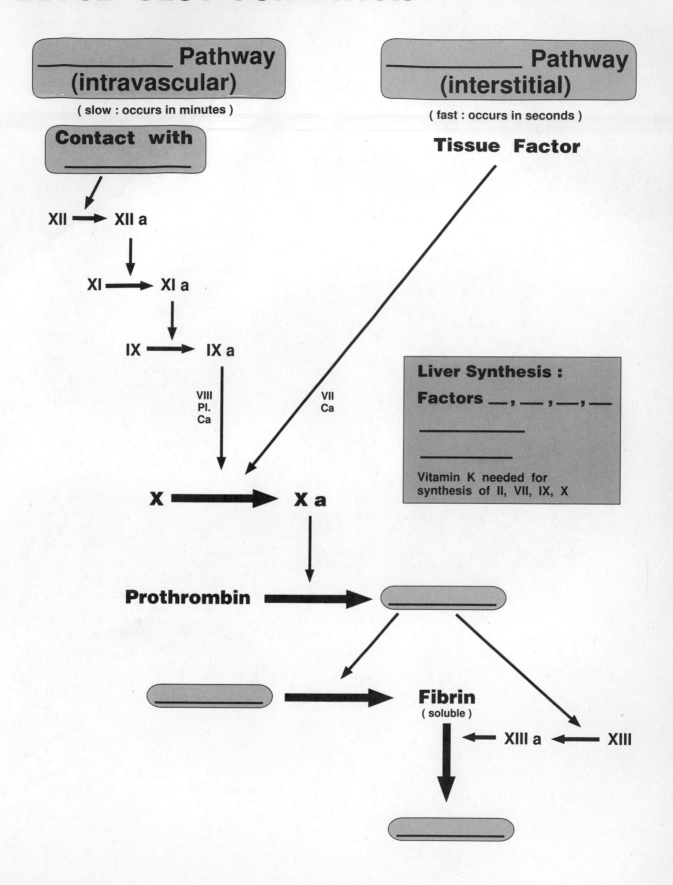

_____ Pathway (intravascular)

(slow : occurs in minutes)

Contact with _____

XII → XII a

XI → XI a

IX → IX a

VIII
Pl.
Ca

_____ Pathway (interstitial)

(fast : occurs in seconds)

Tissue Factor

VII
Ca

Liver Synthesis :

Factors ___ , ___ , ___ , ___

_____

_____

Vitamin K needed for synthesis of II, VII, IX, X

X → X a

Prothrombin → _____

_____ → **Fibrin**
(soluble)

XIII a ← XIII

_____

Part III : Terminology

Pronunciation Guide

Pronunciation Key

Accented Syllables
The strongest accented syllable is in capital letters : dī - ag - NŌ - sis

Secondary accents are indicated by a prime (′) : fiz′ - ē - OL - ō - jē

Vowels
Long vowels are indicated by a horizontal line (macron) above the letter :

ā as in bay   ē as in be   ī as in by   ō as in toe

Short vowels are unmarked :

e as in pet   i as in pit   o as in pot   u as in bud

Other Phonetic Symbols
a as in about   oo as in do   yoo as in cute   oy as in noise

NOTE : Arteries and veins appear in separate lists at the end of this section.

adrenaline   a - DREN - a - lin
adventitia   ad - ven - TISH - ya
afferent   AF - er - ent
agranulocyte   a - GRAN - yoo - lō - sīt′
albumin   al - BYOO - min
aldosterone   al - DA - ster - ōn
anastomoses   a - nas - tō - MŌ - sēs
anastomosis   a - nas - tō - MŌ - sis
anemia   a - NĒ - mē - a
aneurysm   AN - yoo - rizm
angina pectoris   an - JĪ - na PEK - tō - ris
angiotensin   an′ - jē - ō - TEN - sin
angiotensinogen   an′ - jē - ō - TEN - sin - ō - jen
antidiuretic   an′ - ti - dī - yoo - RET - ik
aorta   ā - OR - ta
arteriole   ar - TĒ - rē - ōl
arteriovenous   ar - tē′ - rē - ō - VĒ - nus
artery   AR - ter - ē
atherosclerosis   ath′ - er - ō - skle - RŌ - sis
atria   Ā - trē - a
atrial   Ā - trē - al
atrioventricular   ā - trē - ō - ven - TRIK - yoo - lar
atrium   Ā - trē - um
auscultation   aws - kul - TĀ - shun
auscultatory   aws - KUL - ta - tō′ - rē
azygos   AZ - i - gos

basophil   BĀ - sō - fil
bicuspid   bī - KUS - pid
bifurcate   bī - FUR - kāt
bilirubin   bil - ē - ROO - bin
biliverdin   bil - ē - VER - din
bradycardia   brād′ - i - KAR - dē - a

bundle of His   HISS

capillary   KAP - i - lar′ - ē
cardiology   kar - dē - OL - ō - jē
carotid   ka - ROT - id
cerebrovascular   se - rē - brō - VAS - kyoo - lar
chordae tendineae   KOR - dē ten - DIN - ē - ē
collagen   KOL - a - jen
colloid   KOL - oyd
contractility   kon′ - trak - TIL - i - tē
cytokine   SĪ - tō - kīn
cytotoxic   sī′ - tō - TOK - sik

desmosome   DEZ - mō - sōm
diastole   dī - AS - tō - lē
diastolic   dī - as - TOL - ik

edema   e - DĒ - ma
efferent   EF - er - ent
electrolye   ē - LEK - trō - līt′
embolism   EM - bō - lizm
embolus   EM - bō - lus
eosinophil   ē - ō - SIN - ō - fil
epinephrine   ep - ē - NEF - rin
erythrocyte   e - RITH - rō - sīt′
erythropoiesis   e - rith′ - rō - poy - Ē - sis
erythropoietin   e - rith′ - rō - POY - ē - tin
extrinsic   ek - STRIN - sik

fenestrated   FEN - es - trāt′ - ed
fibrillation   fi - bri - LĀ - shun
fibrin   FĪ - brin
fibrinogen   fī - BRIN - ō - jen

176

fibrinolysis fī - brin - OL - i - sis

gout GOWT
granular GRAN - yoo - lar
granulocyte GRAN - yoo - lō - sīt′

hematocrit hē - MAT - ō - krit
hematology hēm - a - TOL - ō - jē
hematopoiesis hem′ - a - tō - poy - Ē - sis
heme HĒM
hemodynamics hē′ - mō - dī - NA - miks
hemoglobulin HĒ - mō - glō′ - bin
hemolysis hē - MOL - i - sis
hemophilia hē′ - mō - FĒL - ē - a
hemopoiesis hē′ - mō - poy - Ē - sis
hemorrhage HEM - or - rij
hemorrhoid HEM - ō - royd
hemostasis hē′ - mō - STĀ - sis
heparin HEP - a - rin
hepatic he - PAT - ik
histamine HISS - ta - mēn
hypovolemic hī′ - pō - vō - LĒ - mik
hypoxia hī - POKS - ē - a

immunoglobulin im′ - yoo - nō - GLOB - yoo - lin
infarction in - FARK - shun
intercalated in - TER - ka - lāt - ed
interstitial in′ - ter - STISH - al
intrinsic in - TRIN - sik
isovolumetric ī′ - sō - vol - yoo - MET - rik

Korotkoff kō - ROT - kof
Kupffer KOOP - fer

leukemia loo - KĒ - mē - a
leukocyte LOO - kō - sīt
leukocytosis loo′ - kō - sī - TŌ - sis
leukopenia loo - kō - PĒ - nē - a
lipoprotein lip′ - ō - PRŌ - tēn
lumen LOO - men
lymph LIMF
lymphatic lim - FAT - ik
lymphocyte LIM - fō - sīt

macrophage MAK - rō - fāj
mediastinum mē′ - dē - a - STĪ - num
megakaryocyte meg′ - a - KAR - ē - ō - sīt′
metarteriole met′ - ar - TĒ - rē - ōl
monocyte MON - ō - sīt
myocardium mī - ō - KAR - dē - um

natriuretic nā′ - trē - yoo - RET - ik
neutrophil NOO - trō - fil
noradrenaline nor - a - DREN - a - lin

norepinephrine nor′ - ep - ē - NEF - rin

osmoreceptor oz′ - mō - re - CEP - tor
osmosis os - MŌ - sis   oz - MŌ - sis

papilla pa - PIL - a
papillary PAP - i - ler′ - ē
parasympathetic par′ - a - sim - pa - THET - ik
parietal pa - RĪ - e - tal
pericardial per′ - i - KAR - dē - al
pericardium per′ - i - KAR - dē - um
phagocyte FAG - ō - sīt
phagocytosis fag′ - ō - sī - TŌ - sis
phlebitis fle - BĪ - tis
pinocytosis pi′ - nō - sī - TŌ - sis
plaque PLAK
plasma PLAZ - ma
plasmin PLAZ - min
plasminogen plaz - MIN - ō - jen
pluripotent ploo - RIP - ō - tent
prothrombin prō - THROM - bin
pulmonary PUL - mo - ner′ - ē
Purkinje pur - KIN - jē

renin RĒ - nin
reticulocyte re - TIK - yoo - lō - sīt′

sarcolemma sar′ - kō - LEM - ma
semilunar sem′ - ē - LOO - nar
serous SIR - us
serum SĒ - rum
sinoatrial sī - nō - Ā - trē - al
sinus SĪ - nus
sinusoid SĪN - yoo - soyd
sinusoidal SĪN - yoo - soyd - al
sphincter SFINGK - ter
sphygmomanometer sfig′ - mō - ma - NOM - e - ter
spleen SPLĒN
stasis STĀ - sis
stenosis sten - Ō - sis
systemic sis - TEM - ik
systole SIS - tō - lē
systolic sis - TOL - ik

tachycardia tak′ - i - KAR - dē - a
thoracic thō - RAS - ik
thrombin THROM - bin
thrombocyte THROM - bō - sīt
thrombosis throm - BŌ - sis
thrombus THROM - bus
trabeculae carneae tra - BEK - yoo - lē KAR - nē - ē
tricuspid trī - KUS - pid
tunica adventitia TOO - ni - ka ad′ - ven - TISH - ya
tunica externa TOO - ni - ka eks - TER - na

tunica interna   TOO-ni-ka in-TER-na
tunica intima   TOO-ni-ka IN-ti-ma
tunica media   TOO-ni-ka MĒ-dē-a

vas   VAS
vasa vasorum   VA-sa va-SŌ-rum
vascular   VAS-kyoo-lar
vasoconstriction   vas′-ō-kon-STRIK-shun
vasodilation   vas′-ō-dī-LĀ-shun
vasomotion   vas′-ō-MŌ-shun
vasomotor   vas′-ō-MŌ-tor
vasopressin   vas′-ō-PRES-in
vena cava   VĒ-na KĀ-va
venae cavae   VĒ-nē KĀ-vē
venule   VEN-yool
visceral   VIS-er-al
viscosity   vis-KOS-i-tē

Arteries and Veins

The following terms are used for both arteries and veins :

axillary   AK-si-ler′-ē

brachial   BRĀ-kē-al
brachiocephalic   brā-kē-ō-se-FAL-ik
bronchial   BRONG-kē-al

cecal   SĒ-kal
cephalic   se-FAL-ik
cerebral   SER-e-bral (se-RĒ-bral)
circumflex   SER-kum-fleks
colic   KOL-ik
communicating   ko-MYOO-ni-kā-ting
coronary   KOR-o-nar-ē
cystic   SIS-tik

digital   DIJ-i-tal
dorsalis pedis   dor-SA-lis PED-is′

esophageal   e-sof′-a-JĒ-al

femoral   FEM-o-ral

gastric   GAS-trik
gastroepiploic   gas′-trō-ep′-i-PLŌ-ik
gastro-omental   gas′-trō-ō-MEN-tal
gonadal   gō-NAD-al

hepatic   he-PAT-ik

ileal   IL-ē-al
ileocolic   il′-ē-ō-KOL-ik
iliac   IL-ē-ak
intercostal   in′-ter-KOS-tal

jejunal   je-JOO-nal

lumbar   LUM-bar

marginal   MAR-ji-nal
mediastinal   mē′-dē-as-TĪ-nal
mesenteric   MES-en-ter′-ik
metacarpal   met′-a-KAR-pal

ovarian   ō-VA-rē-an

palmar   PAL-mar
pancreatic   pan′-krē-AT-ik
pancreaticoduodenal   pan′-krē-at′-i-kō-doo′-ō-DĒ-nal
pericardial   per′-i-KAR-dē-al
peroneal   per′-ō-NĒ-al
phrenic   FREN-ik
plantar   PLAN-tar
popliteal   pop′-li-TĒ-al
pulmonary   PUL-mo-ner′-ē
pyloric   pī-LOR-ik

radial   RĀ-dē-al
rectal   REK-tal
renal   RĒ-nal

sacral   SĀ-kral
sigmoid   SIG-moyd
splenic   SPLĒN-ik
subclavian   sub-KLĀ-vē-an
subcostal   SUB-kos-tal
suprarenal   soo′-pra-RĒ-nal

testicular   tes-TIK-yoo-lar
tibial   TIB-ē-al

ulnar   UL-nar

vertebral   VER-te-bral

Arteries

The following terms are used for arteries only :

aorta   ā - OR - ta

basilar   BAS - i - lar
brachiocephalic trunk   brā - kē - ō - se - FAL - ik

carotid   ka - ROT - id
celiac trunk   SĒ - lē - ak

gastroduodenal   gas' - trō - doo' - ō - DĒ - nal

interventricular   in' - ter - ven - TRIK - yoo - lar

pulmonary trunk   PUL - mo - ner' - ē

Veins

The following terms are used for veins only :

antebrachial   an' - tē - BRĀ - kē - al
azygos   AZ - i - gos

basilic   ba - SIL - ik

cardiac   KAR - dē - ak
cubital   KYOO - bi - tal

dorsal venous arch   DOR - sal VĒ - nus

hemiazygos   hem' - ē - a - ZĪ - gos
hepatic portal   he - PAT - ik

inferior vena cava   VĒ - na KĀ - va

jugular   JUG - yoo - lar

palmar venous arch   PAL - mar VĒ - nus
plantar venous arch   PLAN - tar VĒ - nus

saphenous   sa - FĒ - nus
vena cava   VĒ - na KĀ - va

venae cavae   VĒ - nē' KĀ - vē'

Venous Sinuses

The following terms are used for venous sinuses :

cavernous   KAV - er - nus
coronary   KOR - o - nar - ē

occipital   ok - SIP - i - tal

sagittal   SAJ - i - tal
sigmoid   SIG - moyd
straight   STRĀT

transverse   trans - VERS

Glossary of Terms

Adrenal cortex   The outer portion of an adrenal gland. It secretes aldosterone, cortisol, and small amounts of sex hormones.

Adrenaline   *See* Epinephrine.

Adrenal medulla   The inner portion of an adrenal gland. It secretes epinephrine and norepinephrine in response to stimulation by preganglionic sympathetic neurons.

Afferent   Carrying toward. Applies to blood vessels and nerves.

Agranular leukocyte   A white blood cell that does not have granules. Includes lymphocytes and monocytes. Also called *agranulocyte*.

Agranulocyte   *See* Agranular leukocyte.

Albumin   The most abundant and smallest of the plasma proteins. Helps to regulate the osmotic pressure of plasma.

Aldosterone   A hormone secreted by the adrenal cortex. It acts on the kidneys, promoting the retention of sodium (and therefore of water) and the excretion of potassium.

Ammonia (NH_3)   A toxic substance produced by cells during the breakdown of amino acids. It is converted into urea by the liver.

Anastomosis   (plural : anastomoses)   A joining together of blood vessels, lymphatic vessels, or nerves.

Anemia   Condition of the blood in which the number of functional red blood cells or their hemoglobin content is below normal.

Aneurysm   A saclike enlargement of a blood vessel caused by a weakening of its wall.

Angina pectoris   Chest pain associated with inadequate blood flow to heart muscle (myocardium).

Angiotensin I   A protein generated in the plasma by the action of the enzyme renin on angiotensinogen.

Angiotensin II   A hormone formed by the action of an ezyme on angiotensin I. It stimulates the adrenal cortex to secrete aldosterone and causes vasoconstriction of blood vessels. Both actions tend to elevate the blood pressure.

Angiotensinogen   Inactive plasma protein that is converted into angiotensin I (by the action of the enzyme renin).

Anterior   Nearer to the front; opposite of posterior. Also called *ventral*.

Antidiuretic hormone (ADH)   A hormone produced by neurosecretory cells in the paraventricular and supraoptic nuclei of the hypothalamus and secreted by the posterior pituitary gland. It promotes the retention of water by the kidneys and vasoconstriction of arterioles. Its actions tend to elevate the blood pressure. Also called *vasopressin*.

Aorta   The largest artery in the body. It carries blood from the left ventricle of the heart, down through the thorax to the abdomen, where it branches into the the right and left common iliac arteries.

Aortic bodies   Chemoreceptors on or near the arch of the aorta. They are sensitive to blood levels of oxygen, carbon dioxide, and hydrogen ions.

Aortic reflex   A reflex concerned with maintaining normal systemic blood pressure.

Aortic valve   The valve between the left ventricle of the heart and the aorta. Also called the *aortic semilunar valve*.

Arteriole   A small (almost microscopic) blood vessel between an artery and capillary. It is surrounded by smooth muscle and is the primary site of vascular resistance; regulates blood distribution.

Arteriovenous anastomosis   A vessel that connects an arteriole directly with a venule, bypassing a capillary bed.

Artery   A thick-walled, elastic blood vessel that carries blood away from the heart to arterioles.

Atherosclerosis   A process in which fatty substances (cholesterol and triglycerides) are deposited in the walls of medium and large arteries.

Atrial contraction   One of the five phases of the cardiac cycle.

Atrial natriuretic peptide (ANP)   A hormone secreted by cardiac muscle fibers of the atria in response to stretching. It increases sodium and water excretion in the urine (natriuresis and diuresis) and causes vasodilation of blood vessels. Both actions tend to decrease the blood pressure. Also called *atrial natriuretic factor (ANF)*.

Atrial reflex   *See* Right heart reflex.

Atrioventricular bundle   The portion of the conduction system of the heart that begins at the AV node, passes through the nonconducting tissue separating the atria and ventricles, then runs a short distance down the interventricular septum before splitting into the right and left bundle branches. Also called the *bundle of His*.

Atrioventricular node (AV node)   A specialized area of small-diameter fibers located at the base of the right atrium near the interventricular septum. To get from the atria into the ventricles electrical impulses must pass through the AV node; the small-diameter fibers slow down the speed of electrical transmission, allowing the atria time to finish contracting before the ventricles begin to contract.

Atrioventricular valve (AV valve)   A valve that permits blood to flow in one direction only: from the atria into the ventricles. The right AV valve is also called the *tricuspid valve*; the left AV valve is also called the *bicuspid valve*.

Atrium   (plural: atria)   A superior chamber of the heart. The right atrium receives deoxygenated blood from the superior and inferior venae cavae; the left atrium receives oxygenated blood from four pulmonary veins.

Auscultation   Examination by listening to sounds in the body.

Auscultatory method   A method of measuring arterial blood pressure, using a sphygmomanometer and stethoscope.

Autoregulation   The ability of an organ to control (self-regulate) blood flow by controlling the lumen diameter (vascular resistance) of arterioles leading to that organ. It depends on tissue needs; it is independent of neural and hormonal influences.

Azygos   An anatomical structure that is not paired; occurring singly.

Bainbridge reflex   The increased heart rate that follows increased pressure or distention of the right atrium.

Baroreceptor   A receptor sensitive to pressure or the rate of change of pressure. Arterial baroreceptors are sensory nerve endings located in the carotid sinuses and the aortic arch; they respond to decreased blood pressure by decreasing their output to the cardiovascular center (in the medulla oblongata). Intrarenal baroreceptors are pressure-sensitive granular cells in the kidneys that respond to decreased renal arterial pressure by secreting renin.

Basement membrane   A thin layer of extracellular material that attaches epithelial tissue to the underlying connective tissue.

Basophil   A type of white blood cell characterized by large granules that stain with basic dyes. They enter tissues and become mast cells, which secrete histamine. Basophils increase during allergic reactions.

B cell   One of the two basic types of lymphocytes (the other type is the T cell). When activated, a B cell develops into a plasma cell, which secretes antibodies.

Bicuspid valve   The atrioventricular valve between the left atrium and left ventricle. Also called the *mitral valve*.

Bifurcate   Having two branches or divisions; forked.

Bilirubin   A red or yellowish pigment resulting from the breakdown of hemoglobin by liver cells. It is excreted as a waste product in the bile (fluid produced by the liver).

Biliverdin   A green pigment resulting from the breakdown of hemoglobin by liver cells. It is excreted as a waste product in the bile (fluid produced by the liver).

Blood   A type of connective tissue. Consists of formed elements (red blood cells, white blood cells, and platelets) and plasma. Also called *vascular tissue*.

Blood capillary   *See* Capillary.

Blood colloid osmotic pressure (BCOP)   The pressure caused by the difference in water concentrations in the plasma and interstitial fluid. It tends to pull water from the interstitial fluid (higher water concentration) into the plasma (lower water concentration). The plasma has a lower water concentration because it has more colloids (large molecules), especially plasma proteins.

Blood hydrostatic pressure (BHP)   The pressure exerted by blood plasma on the walls of a blood vessel. It is determined by the volume of blood and the elasticity of the blood vessel that contains it. Blood hydrostatic pressure causes plasma to filter out of capillaries into the interstitial spaces.

Blood pressure (BP)   *See* Blood hydrostatic pressure (BHP).

Blood reservoirs   Systemic veins and the spleen are called blood reservoirs. They contain large amounts of blood that can be moved quickly to other parts of the body.

Blood type   Blood classification based on the presence or absence of certain proteins on the surfaces of red blood cells. Types A, B, AB, and O; Rh negative and Rh positive.

Blood vessels   Arteries, arterioles, capillaries, venules, and veins.

Bone marrow   Site of erythrocyte, leukocyte, and platelet synthesis. Contains stem cells from which all types of blood cells are derived.

Bradycardia   A slow resting heart rate or pulse rate (under 60/minute).

Buffer   A weak acid or base that can exist in an undissociated form (H-buffer) or in a dissociated form (H^+ + buffer).

Buffer system   A pair of chemicals, a weak acid and a weak base, that minimize changes in the pH (acidity) of a solution when acid is added or removed. An example is the carbonic acid–bicarbonate buffer system: when there is a shortage of hydrogen ions, carbonic acid releases them; when there is an excess of hydrogen ions, bicarbonate combines with them.

Bulk flow   The movement of a fluid (gas or liquid) that results from a hydrostatic pressure gradient. Examples are the flow of blood and the flow of air in and out of the lungs.

Bundle branch   One of the two branches of the atrioventricular bundle. Specialized muscle fibers that transmit electrical impulses very rapidly to the bottom tip of both ventricles, where they divide into smaller fibers called conduction myofibers (Purkinje fibers).

Bundle of His   *See* Atrioventricular bundle.

Capillary   A microscopic blood vessel located between an arteriole and venule. The only location where materials are exchanged between the blood and body cells. Also called *blood capillary*.

Cardiac   Pertaining to the heart.

Cardiac arrest   Cessation of an effective heartbeat.

Cardiac cycle   A complete heartbeat. It may be divided into five phases: isovolumetric relaxation, passive filling, atrial contraction, isovolumetric ventricular contraction, ejection.

Cardiac muscle   The branched, striated muscle fibers that make up the middle layer (myocardium) of the heart wall.

Cardiac output (CO)   The volume of blood pumped from one ventricle in one minute; about 5.2 liters/minute under normal resting conditions. (Not the total output of both ventricles.)

Cardiac reserve   The maximum percentage that cardiac output can increase above normal.

Cardio-accelerator center   Portion of the cardiovascular center containing neurons that stimulate the heart to contract faster and more forcefully (via sympathetic nerves).

Cardio-inhibitory center   Portion of the cardiovascular center containing neurons that slow down the heart rate (via parasympathetic nerves).

Cardiology   The study of the heart and diseases associated with it.

Cardiovascular center   A group of neurons in the medulla oblongata (brain stem) that act as an integrating center for reflexes that regulate heart rate, force of contraction (stroke volume), and blood vessel diameter.

Cardiovascular system   The heart and blood vessels.

Carotid body   Chemoreceptor on or near the carotid sinus that responds to changes in blood levels of oxygen, carbon dioxide, and hydrogen ions.

Carotid sinus   A dilated region of the internal carotid artery just above the bifurcation of the common carotid artery. Contains sensory nerve endings called baroreceptors that monitor blood pressure.

Carotid sinus reflex   A reflex concerned with maintaining normal blood pressure in the brain.

Cascade   A series of reactions in which each reaction is triggered by the preceeding one. Once initiated, it continues to the final reaction. An example is the series of reactions for the formation of a blood clot (the intrinsic and extrinsic clotting pathways).

Cerebral arterial circle   The ring of arteries at the base of the brain between the internal carotid and basilar arteries. Also called the *circle of Willis*.

Cerebrovascular accident   The destruction of brain tissue resulting from occlusion or rupture of cerebral vessels. Also called a *stroke*.

Chemically gated ion channel   An ion channel that opens and closes in response to a specific chemical stimulus, such as a neurotransmitter, hormone, or certain ions.

Chemoreceptor   A sensory nerve ending that is sensitive to the plasma concentrations of certain chemicals, especially oxygen, carbon dioxide, and hydrogen ions. Examples are the carotid and aortic bodies.

Cholesterol   The most abundant steroid (type of lipid) in animal tissues; located in cell membranes and used for the synthesis of steroid hormones and bile salts.

Chordae tendineae   Tendonlike, fibrous cords that connect the atrioventricular valves with the papillary muscles inside the ventricles of the heart. They strengthen the atrioventricular valves, preventing eversion during systole.

Circle of Willis   *See* Cerebral arterial circle.

Clot   The end result of a series of biochemical reactions that change liquid plasma into a gelatinous mass.

Coagulation   The process by which a blood clot is formed.

Collagen   A type of protein fiber found in most types of connective tissues. Gives strength to the walls of blood vessels.

Collateral circulation   The alternate route taken by blood through an anastomosis.

Colloid   A large molecule, mainly protein, suspended in a liquid. Capillaries are relatively impermeable to colloids.

Colony stimulating factor (CSF)   One of a group of hormones that stimulate the development of white blood cells.

Complete blood count (CBC)   A blood test that usually includes hemoglobin determination, hematocrit, red and white blood cell count, differential white blood cell count, and platelet count.

Conduction myofibers   Part of the conduction system of the heart. Specialized muscle fibers that conduct electrical impulses from the right and left bundle branches to the myocardium of the ventricles. Also called Purkinje fibers.

Conduction system   A network of cardiac muscle fibers that are specialized for the generation and distribution of electrical impulses. Structures include the SA node (pacemaker), AV node, AV bundle, right and left bundle branches, and conduction myofibers (Purkinje fibers).

Continuous capillary   A capillary in which the plasma membranes of endothelial cells form a continuous, uninterrupted ring around the capillary. This type of capillary is found in smooth muscle, skeletal muscle, connective tissues, and the lungs.

Contractility   The force of cardiac muscle contraction not due to increased end-diastolic volume.

Coronary   Pertaining to the heart.

Coronary artery disease   A condition such as atherosclerosis that causes narrowing of coronary arteries. As a result, the heart muscle receives inadequate amounts of blood.

Coronary circulation   The pathway followed by the blood from the ascending aorta through the blood vessels supplying the heart (coronary arteries) and returning to the right atrium. Also called the *cardiac circulation*.

Coronary sinus   A wide venous channel on the posterior surface of the heart that collects the blood from the coronary circulation and returns it to the right atrium.

Cytokines   Substances produced by activated lymphocytes and other cells. They have a variety of roles in immunity and blood cell development.

Cytotoxic T cell   A type of T cell that, when activated, directly attacks virus-infected cells and tumor cells.

Depolarization   The process by which a membrane becomes more positive on the inside. It is usually caused by the movement of sodium ions into the cell.

Desmosome   A type of cell junction that holds adjacent cells firmly together. Found in tissues that are subject to considerable stretching, such as the cardiac muscle cells. Desmosomes may be compared to rivets that link cells together.

Diastole   The relaxation phase of the cardiac cycle. The period of time when the ventricles are not contracting.

Diastolic blood pressure (DBP)   The lowest blood pressure measured in large arteries. Under normal conditions, about 80 mm Hg for a young adult male.

Differential white blood cell count   Determination of the number of each kind of white blood cell in a sample of 100 cells for diagnostic purposes.

Diffusion   A passive process in which there is a net movement of molecules or ions from a region of high concentration to a region of low concentration until equilibrium is reached.

Dorsal   Nearer to the back; opposite of ventral. Refers to the back of the hand (opposite of palmar) and the top of the foot (opposite of plantar). Also called *posterior*.

ECG   *See* Electrocardiogram.

Edema   An abnormal accumulation of interstitial fluid.

Efferent   Carrying away from. Applies to blood vessels and nerves.

EKG   *See* Electrocardiogram.

Elastic arteries   Large arteries with lumen diameters of between 1 and 2 cm. They have a larger percentage of elastin fibers than smaller arteries. Also called *conducting arteries*.

Electrocardiogram (ECG or EKG)   A recording of the electrical changes that accompany the cardiac cycle. They can be recorded on the surface of the skin. Electrocardiograms may be resting, stress, or ambulatory.

Electrolyte   Any compound that separates (dissociates) into ions when dissolved in water.

Embolism   The obstruction or closure of a blood vessel by an embolus.

Embolus   A blood clot, bubble of air, fat from broken bones, mass of bacteria, or other debris or foreign material transported by the blood.

End-diastolic volume (EDV)   The volume of blood, remaining in a ventricle at the end of its relaxation phase (just before ventricular contraction begins). At rest, it is about 130 ml.

Endocardium   The inner lining of the heart. It consists of endothelial cells and is continuous with the lining of the great vessels attached to the heart.

Endothelium   The layer of simple squamous epithelium that lines the cavities of the heart, blood vessels, and lymphatic vessels.

End-systolic volume (ESV)   The volume of blood remaining in a ventricle following its contraction. At rest, the ESV is about 60 ml.

Eosinophil   A type of white blood cell involved in allergic responses and the destruction of parasitic worms. It is characterized by granular cytoplasm readily stained by a red dye called eosin.

Epicardium   The thin, transparent membrane surrounding the heart. Also called the *visceral pericardium*.

Epinephrine   A hormone secreted by the adrenal medulla. Its actions are similar to those that result from sympathetic stimulation; it increases heart rate and force of contraction (stroke volume). Also called *adrenaline*.

Erythrocyte   A cell with no nucleus that has the shape of a biconcave disc and is filled with hemoglobin. Its function is to transport gases (oxygen and carbon dioxide) in the blood between the lungs and tissue cells. Also called a *red blood cell (RBC)*.

Erythropoiesis   The process by which erythrocytes are formed in the bone marrow.

Erythropoietin   A hormone released by the kidneys and liver in response to low blood oxygen concentrations. It stimulates increased production of erythrocytes (red blood cells) in the the bone marrow.

Eversion   The movement of the sole outward at the ankle joint or of an atrioventricular valve (bicuspid or tricuspid valve) into an atrium during ventricular contraction.

Excitability   The ability of muscle and nerve cells to produce electrical signals (action potentials) in response to stimuli.

Extracellular fluid (ECF)   Fluid outside the cells. Includes blood plasma and interstitial fluid.

Extrinsic   Coming from outside.

Extrinsic clotting pathway   The cascade of reactions leading to blood clotting that is initiated by the release of a substance called tissue factor from damaged blood vessels or surrounding tissues.

Factor XII   The initial factor in the intrinsic clotting pathway. It is activated by contact with the collagen exposed when blood vessel linings are damaged. Also called *Hageman factor*.

Fenestrated capillary   Capillaries in which the endothelial cells appear to be perforated. These perforations (fenestrations or "little windows") allow for more rapid exchange of materials between blood and the tissues.

Fibrillation   Rapid, unsynchronized cardiac muscle contractions; prevents the effective pumping of blood.

Fibrin   A protein formed from fibrinogen by the action of thrombin.

Fibrinogen   The plasma protein precursor of fibrin.

Fibrinolysis   The dissolution of a blood clot by the action of an enzyme that converts insoluble fibrin into a soluble substance.

Fibrous pericardium   The tough, outer layer of the double-layered membrane that surrounds the heart. It protects the heart from overdistension during vigorous exercise.

Fick method   A method for measuring the cardiac output.

Filtration   The movement of plasma (minus most of the plasma proteins) across capillary walls into the interstitial spaces.

Flow (of blood)   The volume of blood flow between any two points in the cardiovascular system is directly proportional to the pressure difference between the points and inversely proportional to the resistance.

Formed elements   Red blood cells, white blood cells, and platelets.

Gamma globulin (IgG)   *See* Immunoglobulin.

Gap junction   A type of cell junction that consists of small channels filled with cytoplasm connecting adjacent cells. A gap junction allows ions and small molecules to flow between adjacent cells; it facilitates the transmission of electrical signals between heart muscle cells.

Gout   Hereditary condition associated with excessive uric acid in the blood; the acid crystallizes and deposits in joints, kidneys, and soft tissues.

Granular leukocyte   Neutrophils, eosinophils, and basophils. White blood cells that have granules in their cytoplasm. Also called *granulocyte*.

Granulocyte   *See* Granular leukocyte.

Great arteries   The pulmonary trunk and aorta. Large arteries that emerge from the right and left ventricles of the heart.

Hageman factor   *See* Factor XII.

HDL   *See* High-density lipoprotein.

Heart attack   Damage to or death of cardiac muscle. Also called a *myocardial infarction*.

Heart block   An arrhythmia of the heart in which the atria and ventricles contract independently because of a blocking of electrical impulses at a critical point in the conduction system.

Heart-lung machine   A device that pumps blood, functioning as a heart, and removes carbon dioxide from blood and oxygenates it, functioning as lungs.

Heart murmur   An abnormal heart sound caused by turbulent blood flow through a narrowed or leaky valve (or through a hole in the interventricular or interatrial septum).

Heart rate   The number of heart contractions per minute.

Heart sound   Sounds that can be heard using a stethoscope. They are caused by the vibrations due to the closing of the AV valves (1st heart sound) or the closing of the pulmonary and aortic valves (2nd heart sound).

Heart wall   Three tissue layers that surround the heart: the epicardium (outer layer), myocardium (middle layer), and endocardium (inner layer).

Helper T cell   A type of T cell (lymphocyte) that helps to activate B cells, cytotoxic T cells, and NK cells.

Hematocrit   The percentage of blood occupied by red blood cells. Average values: males 47%; females 42%.

Hematology   The study of blood.

Hematopoiesis   *See* Hemopoiesis.

Heme   An iron-containing organic molecule. Each hemoglobin molecule contains 4 heme groups; each heme group contains one iron atom which binds one oxygen molecule.

Hemodynamics   The study of factors and forces that govern the flow of blood through blood vessels.

Hemoglobin (Hb)   A substance in red blood cells consisting of four polypeptide chains and the iron-containing red pigment heme. About 33% of the red blood cell volume is occupied by hemoglobin; it is involved in the transport of oxygen and carbon dioxide.

Hemolysis   The escape of hemoglobin from the interior of a red blood cell into the surrounding medium.

Hemophilia   A hereditary disorder in which there is a deficient production of certain clotting factors, resulting in excessive bleeding.

Hemopoiesis   Blood cell production; occurs in the red bone marrow of bones. Also called *hematopoiesis*.

Hemorrhage   Bleeding; the escape of blood from blood vessels, especially when it is profuse.

Hemorrhoids   Dilated or varicosed blood vessels (usually veins) in the anal regions. Also called *piles*.

Hemostasis   The stoppage of bleeding.

184

Heparin　An anticlotting agent (anticoagulant) produced by mast cells and basophils. A similar molecule protrudes into the blood from the plasma membranes of endothelial cells.

Hepatic　Pertaining to the liver.

Hepatic portal circulation　The flow of blood from capillaries in the intestines, stomach, spleen, and pancreas to capillaries in the liver.

Hg　The symbol for mercury. Used for measuring pressure in millimeters of mercury (mm Hg).

High-density lipoprotein (HDL)　A type of lipoprotein that removes excess cholesterol from body cells and transports it to the liver for elimination. A high HDL level is associated with decreased risk of heart disease caused by plaque formation. Over 40 mg/dl is desirable.

Histamine　A substance found in many cells, especially mast cells, basophils, and platelets. It is released when cells are injured, causing vasodilation of local arterioles and increased permeability of capillaries (in the lungs it causes constriction of the airways or bronchioles).

Hypertension　Chronic high blood pressure.

Hypovolemic shock　A type of shock characterized by decreased blood volume. It may be caused by acute hemorrhage or excessive fluid loss.

Hypoxia　Lack of adequate oxygen at the tissue level.

Immunoglobulin (Ig)　A synonym for antibody. There are five classes: IgA, IgD, IgE, IgG, and IgM.

Infarction　A localized area of necrotic (dead) tissue produced by inadequate oxygen supply (hypoxia).

Inferior vena cava (IVC)　Large vein that collects blood from parts of the body inferior to the heart; empties into the right atrium.

Inflammation　Localized response to tissue injury. Destroys, dilates, or walls off an infecting agent or injured tissue. Characterized by redness, pain, heat, swelling, and sometimes loss of function.

Intercalated disc　The thickened end of a cardiac muscle cell. Contains desmosomes that hold cardiac cells together and gap junctions that aid in the transmission of muscle action potentials between cells.

Intercellular cleft　The narrow space between adjacent endothelial cells in a capillary. Plasma filters through intercellular clefts into the interstitial spaces.

Intercellular fluid　See Interstitial fluid.

Intercostal　Between the ribs.

Interstitial fluid　The portion of extracellular fluid that fills the microscopic spaces between the cells of tissues. Also called the *intercellular fluid* and *tissue fluid*.

Interstitial fluid osmotic pressure (IFOP)　The osmotic pressure that tends to move fluid out of the capillaries into the interstitial fluid. Compared to the blood colloid osmotic pressure (BCOP), the IFOP is relatively small: 1 mm Hg.

Intrinsic　Of internal origin.

Intrinsic clotting pathway　The cascade of reactions leading to blood clotting that is initiated by contact between collagen and coagulation factor XII.

Ion　Any atom or small molecule that has a net positive or negative charge.

Isovolumetric　Equal (same) volume.

Isovolumetric ventricular contraction　Early phase of systole when the ventricular volume does not change. There is contraction of the ventricles, but no emptying, and there is a rapid rise in the ventricular pressure.

Isovolumetric ventricular relaxation　Early phase of diastole when the ventricular volume does not change. There is relaxation of the ventricles, but no filling; the ventricular pressure is greater than the atrial pressure, so the AV valves remain closed.

Kidney　One of the paired reddish organs located in the lumbar region that regulates the composition and volume of blood and produces urine.

Korotkoff sounds　The various sounds that are heard through a stethoscope, while taking blood pressure.

Kupffer cell　*See* Stellate reticuloendothelial cell.

LDL　*See* Low-density lipoprotein.

Leukemia　A malignant disease of the blood-forming tissues. Characterized by either uncontrolled production and accumulation of immature leukocytes in which many cells fail to reach maturity or an accumulation of mature leukocytes in the blood, because they do not die at the end of their normal life span.

Leukocyte　A white blood cell (WBC). There are five types of leukocytes: neutrophils, eosinophils, basophils, lymphocytes, and monocytes.

Leukocytosis　An increase in the number of white blood cells. Characteristic of many infections and other disorders.

Leukopenia　A decrease in the number of white blood cells (below 5,000/mm^3).

Lipid　An organic molecule composed of carbon, hydrogen, and oxygen. Characterized by insolubility in water. Examples include triglycerides, phospholipids, steroids, and prostaglandins.

Lipid profile　Blood test that measures total cholesterol, high-density lipoprotein, low-density lipoprotein, and triglycerides to assess risk for cardiovascular disease.

Lipoproteins　A lipid that is partially coated by protein. It is produced by the liver and combines with cholesterol and triglycerides to make it water-soluble for transport in the blood.

Low-density lipoprotein (LDL)　Lipoproteins that deliver cholesterol to body cells; they also deposit cholesterol in and around smooth muscle fibers in arteries. High levels of LDL are associated with increased risk of atherosclerosis. Lower than 130 mg/dl is desirable.

Lumbar　Region of the back and side between the ribs and pelvis; loin.

Lumen　The space within an artery, vein, intestine, or a tube.

Lymph　The name given to interstitial fluid when it is inside lymphatic vessels.

Lymphatic capillary　A closed-ended (blind-ended) microscopic lymphatic vessel; it begins in spaces between cells and converges with other lymphatic capillaries to form lymphatic vessels.

Lymphatic system　Includes lymphatic vessels, primary lymphatic organs (bone marrow and thymus gland), secondary lymphatic organs (lymph nodes and spleen), and diffuse lymphatic tissue (tonsils and Peyer's patches).

Lymphatic tissue　A specialized form of reticular connective tissue that contains large numbers of lymphocytes.

Lymphatic vessels　The vessels that carry lymph to the subclavian veins. Includes lymphatic capillaries, lymphatic vessels, lymph trunks, and lymphatic ducts.

Lymph node   An oval or bean-shaped structure located along lymphatic vessels. It contains macrophages, dendritic cells, plasma cells, and lymphocytes (B cells and T cells).

Lymphocyte   The type of leukocyte (white blood cell) responsible for specific (immune) responses. There are two basic types of lymphocytes: B cells and T cells.

Macrophage   A phagocytic cell derived from a monocyte (type of white blood cell).

Mast cell   A cell derived from a basophil (type of white blood cell). Releases histamine and other chemicals involved in inflammation.

Mean arterial blood pressure (MABP)   Average blood pressure during the cardiac cycle. Approximately equal to diastolic pressure plus 1/3 pulse pressure.

Medulla oblongata   The most inferior part of the brain stem; contains the cardiovascular center, which regulates cardiac output and blood pressure.

Megakaryocyte   A large cell in the bone marrow that gives rise to platelets.

Metarteriole   A blood vessel that directly connects an arteriole and venule, bypassing a capillary network.

Microcirculation   Arterioles, capillaries, and venules.

Mitral valve   *See* Bicuspid valve.

Monocyte   The largest of the leukocytes (white blood cells); characterized by agranular cytoplasm. Monocytes leave the bloodstream and are tranformed into macrophages.

Muscle action potential   A change in the membrane potential in the plasma membrane (sarcolemma) of a muscle cell that triggers contraction.

Muscular arteries   Medium-sized arteries with lumen diameters of between 0.1 cm and 1.0 cm. They have a larger percentage of smooth muscle fibers than the larger elastic arteries. Also called *distributing arteries*.

Myocardial infarction   Gross necrosis of myocardial tissue due to interrupted blood supply. Also called a *heart attack*.

Myocardium   The middle layer of the heart wall. Consists of cardiac muscle tissue.

Myogram   The record or tracing produced by the myograph, the apparatus that measures and records the effects of muscular contractions.

Net filtration pressure (NFP)   Net pressure that is used to show the direction of fluid movement in or out of a capillary. Whether fluids leave or enter capillaries depends on how the hydrostatic and osmotic pressures relate to each other.

Neutrophil   The most abundant type of white blood cell; characterized by granular cytoplasm. A phagocytic cell; the first type of cell to appear at the site of an infection.

Noradrenaline   *See* Norepinephrine.

Norepinephrine (NE)   A hormone secreted by the adrenal medulla. It is also secreted by most postganglionic sympathetic nerve fibers. It increases the rate and force of heart contractions and causes vasoconstriction of most blood vessels; increases cardiac output and blood pressure. Also called *noradrenaline*.

Occlusion   The act of closure or state of being closed.

Osmoreceptor   A receptor in the hypothalamus that is sensitive to changes in blood osmotic pressure (BOP). In response to high BOP (low water concentration), it stimulates the release of antidiuretic hormone (ADH) from the posterior pituitary gland. (ADH promotes retention of water by the kidneys and causes vasoconstriction.)

Osmosis   The net diffusion of water molecules through a selectively permeable membrane.

Osmotic pressure   The pressure required to prevent the movement of pure water through a selectively permeable membrane into a solution containing solutes.

Pacemaker   *See* Sinoatrial node.

Palmar   Refers to the palm of the hand. Opposite of dorsal.

Papilla   A small nipple-shaped projection or elevation.

Papillary muscle   Muscles located on the inner surfaces of the ventricles that regulate the tension in the chordae tendineae. They prevent the AV valves from everting into the atria during systole.

Parasympathetic nerves   Autonomic nerves whose postganglionic fibers release acetylcholine (ACh). Parasympathetic stimulation slows down the heart rate.

Pericardial cavity   A space between the parietal and visceral layers of the serous pericardium; it contains a thin film of serous fluid that holds the two layers together.

Pericardium   Connective tissue sac that encloses the heart. Consists of an outer fibrous pericardium and an inner serous pericardium. The serous pericardium has two layers: the outer parietal layer and the inner visceral layer.

pH   A symbol for the concentration of hydrogen ions (H^+) in solution; the acidity of the solution.

Phagocyte   A cell capable of ingesting and destroying particulate matter. There are two major types of phagocytic cells: neutrophils and macrophages.

Phagocytosis   The process by which cells (phagocytes) ingest microbes, worn-out or damaged tissue cells, and other particulate matter.

Phlebitis   Inflammation of a vein, usually in the lower extremities.

Pinocytosis   The process by which cells ingest liquids.

Plantar   Refers to the sole of the foot. Opposite of dorsal.

Plaque   A mass within an artery that causes the inner surface to bulge into the lumen, obstructing the flow of blood. It is composed of cholesterol, smooth muscle cells, collagen, cell debris, and calcium (in older persons).

Plasma   Blood minus the formed elements. The liquid portion of blood.

Plasma cell   A cell that produces antibodies. Develops from an activated B cell (a type of lymphocyte).

Plasma proteins   Proteins present in blood that are not used as nutrients. The three main types are albumins, globulins, and fibrinogen.

Plasmin   An enzyme able to decompose fibrin; it dissolves blood clots.

Plasminogen   Inactive precursor of plasmin.

Platelet   *See* Thrombocyte.

Platelet plug   Aggregation of platelets (thrombocytes) at a damaged blood vessel to prevent blood loss.

Pluripotent hematopoietic stem cells   A population of stem cells found in bone marrow from which all blood cells are descended. Previously called *hemocytoblast*.

Portal vessel   Blood vessel that links two capillary networks.

Examples include the hypophyseal portal veins that carry blood from the hypothalamus to the anterior pituitary gland and the hepatic portal system that carries blood from organs of the digestive tract to the liver.

Posterior   Nearer to the back; opposite of anterior. Also called *dorsal*.

Precapillary sphincter   A ring of smooth muscle around a capillary where it exits from a thoroughfare channel or arteriole. Opens and closes capillaries, regulating blood flow to specific regions of the capillary bed.

Prothrombin   The inactive precursor of thrombin. It is synthesized by the liver, released into the blood, and converted into thrombin in the process of blood clotting.

Pulmonary   Pertaining to the lungs.

Pulmonary circulation   Circulation of blood through the lungs. The flow of deoxygenated blood from the right ventricle to the lungs via the pulmonary trunk and pulmonary arteries; the flow of oxygenated blood from the lungs via the pulmonary veins to the left atrium.

Pulmonary edema   An abnormal accumulation of interstitial fluid in the tissue spaces and alveoli (air sacs) of the lungs.

Pulmonary trunk   The large artery that carries deoxygenated blood out of the right ventricle. It branches into pulmonary arteries that carry the blood to the lungs.

Pulmonary valve   One-way valve between the right ventricle and pulmonary trunk. Also called the *pulmonary semilunar valve*.

Pulmonary veins   Veins that carry oxygenated blood from the lungs to the left atrium.

Pulse pressure   The difference between the maximum (systolic) and minimum (diastolic) pressures. Normally a value of about 40 mm Hg.

Purkinje fibers   *See* Conduction myofibers.

P wave   The deflection wave of an electrocardiogram that records atrial depolarization.

QRS complex   The deflection wave of an electrocardiogrm that records ventricular depolarization.

Red blood cell (RBC)   *See* Erythrocyte.

Refractory period   A period of time during which an excitable cell (muscle or nerve cell) cannot respond to a stimulus that is usually adequate to evoke an action potential.

Renin   An enzyme released by the kidneys into the plasma where it converts angiotensinogen into angiotensin I.

Repolarization   The return of a membrane potential to its resting level.

Residual volume   The volume of blood remaining in a ventricle immediately after systole (contraction).

Resistance   Hindrance to the movement of blood through a vessel. Resistance is directly proportional to the viscosity (thickness) of the blood and the length of the tube; it is inversely proportional to the lumen diameter to the 4th power.

Respiratory pump   The effect of breathing on the movement of blood through the veins (venous return). Changes in intrathoracic and intra-abdominal pressures during inspiration and expiration squeeze blood toward the heart.

Reticulocyte   An immature red blood cell.

Rh factor   An inherited protein (agglutinogen) on the surface of red blood cells. If a person's red blood cells have the Rh factor, they are said to be Rh positive (Rh +); if person's red blood cells do not have the Rh factor, they are said to be Rh negative (Rh −).

Right heart reflex   A reflex concerned with maintaining normal venous blood pressure. Also called the *atrial reflex*.

Sarcolemma   The plasma membrane of a muscle fiber.

Semilunar valve (SL valve)   Valve consisting of three semilunar cusps (half-moon or crescent-shaped flaps of tissue). It permits blood to flow in one direction only: from a ventricle into a great artery (aorta or pulmonary trunk).

Serous pericardium   The inner membrane of the pericardium. It consists of two layers: the outer parietal layer is fused to the fibrous pericardium; the inner visceral layer adheres tightly to the myocardium (muscle of the heart). The visceral layer is also called the epicardium.

Serum   Blood plasma minus fibrinogen and other clotting factors.

Shock   Failure of the cardiovascular system to deliver adequate amounts of oxygen and nutrients to meet the metabolic needs of the body. It is characterized by hypotension (low blood pressure); clammy, cool, pale skin; sweating; reduced urine formation; altered mental state; acidosis; tachychardia (abnormally rapid heartbeat); weak, rapid pulse; and thirst.

Sinoatrial node (SA node)   A mass of cardiac muscle fibers located in the right atrium beneath the opening of the superior vena cava. It determines the heart rate because it spontaneously depolarizes faster than other heart muscle cells. Also called the *pacemaker*.

Sinusoidal capillary   A type of capillary that has a larger diameter than other capillaries and wide spaces between the endothelial cells. Found in certain organs such as the liver and spleen. Also called *sinusoid*.

Sinusoid   *See* Sinusoidal capillary.

Skeletal muscle pump   The effect of contracting skeletal muscles on the movement of blood through the veins (venous return). Contracting muscles bulge and press against nearby veins, squeezing blood toward the heart.

Sphincter   A circular muscle surrounding an opening; contraction of the muscle closes the opening.

Sphygmomanometer   An instrument for measuring arterial blood pressure; consists of an inflatable cuff and a pressure gauge.

Spleen   The largest lymphatic organ; located between the stomach and the diaphragm. It contains macrophages, dendritic cells, plasma cells, and lymphocytes (B cells and T cells).

Starling's law of the heart   Within physiological limits, the greater the length of stretched cardiac muscle fibers, the stronger the contraction. In other words, an increased end-diastolic volume results in an increased stroke volume.

Stasis   Stagnation or halt of normal flow. This pertains to blood, urine, or the contents of the digestive tract.

Stellate reticuloendothelial cell   A phagocytic cell that lines a sinusoid of the liver. Also called a *Kupffer cell*.

Stenosis   An abnormal narrowing or constriction of a duct or opening.

Stethoscope   An instrument for listening to sounds inside the body, such as heart sounds.

Stroke   *See* Cerebrovascular accident.

Stroke volume (SV)   The volume of blood ejected by one

ventricle during one contraction.

Superior vena cava (SVC) Large vein that collects blood from parts of the body superior to the heart; empties into the right atrium.

Suppressor T cell A type of T cell that inhibits antibody production and cytotoxic T cell function.

Sympathetic nerves Autonomic nerves whose postganglionic fibers usually release norepinephrine. Sympathetic stimulation increases the heart rate and stroke volume; it also causes vasoconstriction of blood vessels.

Systemic Affecting the whole body; generalized.

Systemic circulation The circulation of the blood from the left ventricle, through all the organs (except the lungs), and back to the right atrium.

Systemic vascular resistance (SVR) All of the resistance to flow offered by the systemic blood vessels. The major factor controlling the SVR is the diameter of the arterioles. Also called the *total peripheral resistance (TPR)*.

Systole In the cardiac cycle, the period of ventricular contraction.

Systolic blood pressure (SBP) The highest pressure measured in the large arteries. At rest, about 120 mm Hg for a young, adult male.

Tachycardia An abnormally rapid resting heartbeat or pulse rate; over 100 beats/minute.

T cell A lymphocyte (white blood cell) that can differentiate into one of four kinds of cells: helper T cell, cytotoxic T cell, suppressor T cell, and memory T cell. Maturation occurs in the thymus gland.

Thoracic cavity The superior component of the ventral body cavity; between the neck and the diaphragm.

Thoracic duct The main lymphatic vessel. It drains lymph from: the left side of the head, neck, and chest; the left arm; and the entire body below the ribs. It empties into the left subclavian vein. Also called the *left lymphatic duct*.

Thrombin The enzyme that catalyzes the conversion of fibrinogen into fibrin.

Thrombocyte A fragment of cytoplasm enclosed in a cell membrane. Plays a role in blood clotting. Also called a *platelet*.

Thrombosis The formation of a clot (thrombus) in an unbroken blood vessel, usually a vein.

Thrombus A clot formed in an unbroken blood vessel, usually a vein.

Tissue factor (TF) A tissue protein that leaks into the blood from cells outside the the blood vessels. It initiates the extrinsic clotting pathway. Also called *thromboplastin* or *coagulation factor III*.

Total peripheral resistance (TPR) *See* Systemic vascular resistance.

Trabeculae carneae Ridges and folds of the myocardium in the ventricles of the heart.

Transfusion Transfer of whole blood, blood components, or bone marrow directly into the bloodstream.

Tricuspid valve The right atrioventricular valve (AV valve); located between the right atrium and right ventricle.

Tunica externa The outer coat of an artery or vein; composed mostly of collagen fibers. Also called the *tunica adventitia*.

Tunica interna The inner coat of an artery or vein; composed of a lining of endothelium with some collagen fibers. Also called the *tunica intima*.

Tunica media The middle coat of an artery or vein; composed of smooth muscle and elastic fibers.

T wave The deflection wave of an electrocardiogram that respresents ventricular repolarization.

Valvular stenosis A narrowing of a heart valve; usually the bicuspid valve (mitral valve) that is located between the left atrium and left ventricle.

Vas A vessel or duct.

Vasa vasorum Blood vessels that supply nutrients to the larger arteries and veins.

Vascular Pertaining to or containing many blood vessels.

Vascular sinus A channel for blood.

Vascular spasm Contraction of the smooth muscle in the wall of a damaged blood vessel to prevent blood loss.

Vasoconstriction A decrease in blood vessel diameter caused by contraction of the smooth muscle in the wall of the vessel.

Vasodilation An increase in blood vessel diameter caused by relaxation of the smooth muscle in the wall of the vessel.

Vasomotion Intermittent contraction and relaxation of the smooth muscle of the metarterioles and precapillary sphincters that result in an intermittent blood flow.

Vasomotor center A cluster of neurons in the medulla that controls the diameter of blood vessels.

Vasopressin *See* Antidiuretic hormone.

Vein A thin-walled, elastic blood vessel that carries blood toward the heart from the tissues.

Vena cava (plural: venae cavae) One of two large veins that empties deoxygenated blood into the right atrium.

Venous Pertaining to the veins.

Venous return (VR) The volume of blood flowing into the right atrium per minute.

Ventral Nearer to the front; opposite of dorsal. Also called *anterior*.

Ventricle An inferior chamber of the heart. (Also a cavity in the brain.)

Ventricular fibrillation Asynchronous ventricular contractions that result in cardiovascular failure.

Venule A small vein that collects blood from capillaries and delivers it to a vein.

Very low-density lipoprotein (VLDL) Lipoproteins that transport triglycerides synthesized by liver cells to adipose cells for storage. A high-fat diet promotes the production of VLDLs.

Viscosity A property of fluids that determines its resistance to flow.

VLDL *See* Very low-density lipoprotein.

Voltage-sensitive ion channel A plasma membrane ion channel that is opened or closed in response to a change in the membrane potential.

White blood cell (WBC) *See* Leukocyte.

Bibliography

Dorland, William Alexander.   *Dorland's Illustrated Medical Dictionary,* 27th ed.
Philadelphia : W. B. Saunders, 1988.

Fowler, Ira.   *Human Anatomy.*
Belmont, California : Wadsworth, 1984.

Ganong, William F.   *Review of Medical Physiology,* 15th ed.
Norwalk, Connecticut : Appleton & Lange, 1991.

Goldberg, Stephen.   *Clinical Anatomy Made Ridiculously Simple.*
Miami, Florida : MedMaster, 1984.

Junqueira, L. Carlos, Jose Carneiro, and Robert O. Kelley.   *Basic Histology,* 6th ed.
Norwalk, Connecticut : Appleton & Lange, 1989.

Kapit, Wynn and Lawrence M. Elson.   *The Anatomy Coloring Book.*
New York : Harper & Row, 1977.

Melloni, B. J., Ida Dox, and Gilbert Eisner.   *Melloni's Illustrated Medical Dictionary,* 2nd ed.
Baltimore : Williams & Wilkins, 1985.

Moore, Keith L.   *Clinically Oriented Anatomy,* 3rd ed.
Baltimore : Williams & Wilkins, 1992.

Netter, Frank H.   *Atlas of Human Anatomy.*
Summit, New Jersey : Ciba-Geigy, 1989.

Tortora, Gerard J. and Sandra Reynolds Grabowski. *Principles of Anatomy and Physiology,* 7th ed.
New York : HarperCollins, 1993.

Vander, Arthur J., James H. Sherman, and Dorothy S. Luciano.   *Human Physiology,* 5th ed.
New York : McGraw-Hill, 1990.